CHAPTER 1: MEET THE LITTLE JACK

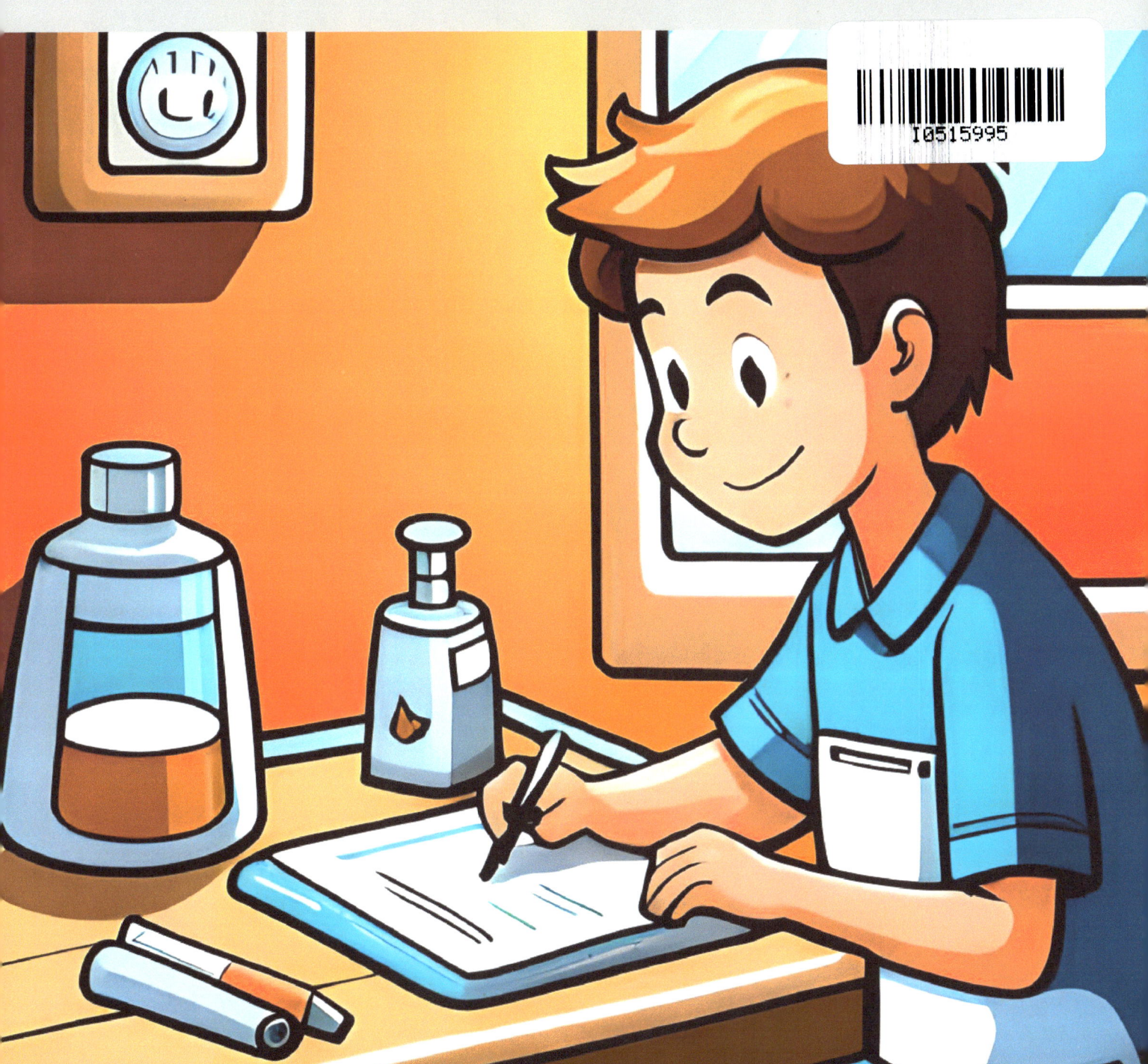

Once upon a time, there was a little boy named Jack who loved animals more than anything else in the world. He had a dog named Max, a cat named Luna, and a parrot named Polly. Jack would spend hours playing with them, petting them, and talking to them as if they were his best friends.

One day, Jack's dog Max got sick, and Jack was really worried. He didn't know what to do, so he asked his mom to take Max to the vet. At the vet clinic, Jack was amazed by all the different animals there – cats, dogs, birds, even a turtle! He watched as the vet examined Max and gave him medicine to help him feel better. Jack was fascinated by how the vet knew exactly what to do to make Max better.

After that day, Jack decided he wanted to become a veterinarian when he grew up. He read books about animals, watched videos about veterinary medicine, and even started a journal to keep track of all the animals he saw and what he learned about them.

Jack's passion for animals grew stronger every day, and he knew that he wanted to spend his life helping animals in need. He dreamed of one day owning his own animal hospital, where he could take care of all kinds of animals and make them feel better. The little veterinarian was born!

ONCE UPON A TIME, IN A FAR-OFF LAND,
THERE LIVED A KING WHO LOVED TO GRANDSTAND.
WITH A VOICE SO BOOMING AND A HEART SO TRUE,
HE RULED HIS KINGDOM AND HIS PEOPLE TOO.

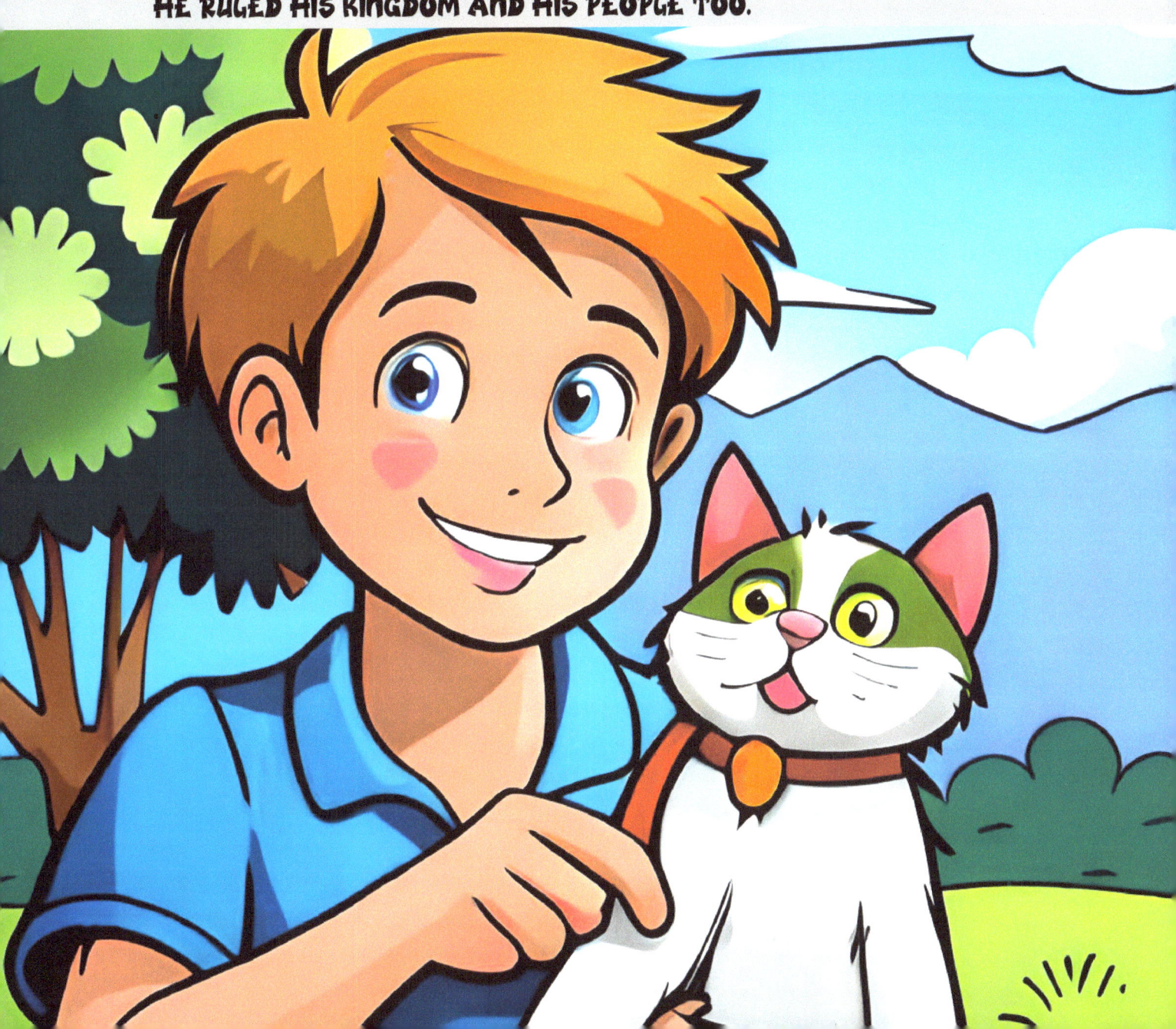

HE WOKE UP EVERY DAY AT DAWN,
AND GREETED THE SUN WITH A ROYAL YAWN.
HE WOULD STRETCH AND DANCE AND SING,
AS THE BIRDS CHIRPED AND THE BELLS DID RING

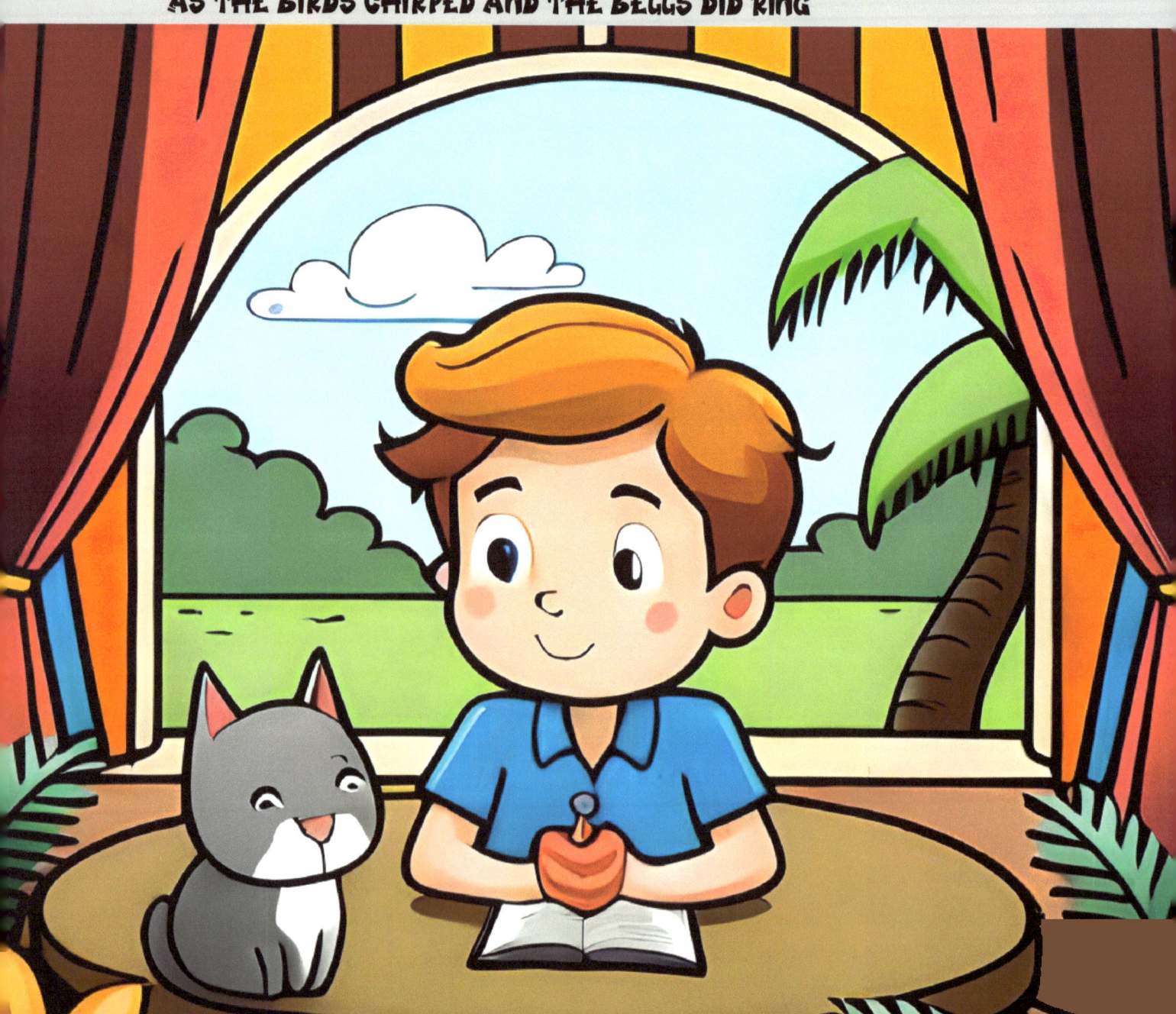

His people loved him, far and wide,
And followed him wherever he would stride.
For his words were like music, sweet and clear,
And his laughter brought joy to all who were near.

One day, the king decided to hold a feast,
And invited all the creatures, from the greatest to the least.
The tables were set, the music did play,
And the king danced with his people, all night and all day.

The rhythm was infectious, and the king led the way,
As the people followed, with their feet in sway.
The animals joined in, with a hop and a skip,
And the birds sang along, with a melody so hip.

The king was in his element, with a smile so wide,
As he danced with his people, side by side.
For he knew that in this moment, he had found the key,
To happiness and joy, for his people and for he.

And so, the king ruled with a rhythm in his heart,
And his people loved him, from the very start.
For he knew that in music, and in dance,
He could bring his people together, in a harmonious trance.

CHAPTER 2: A VISIT TO THE VET

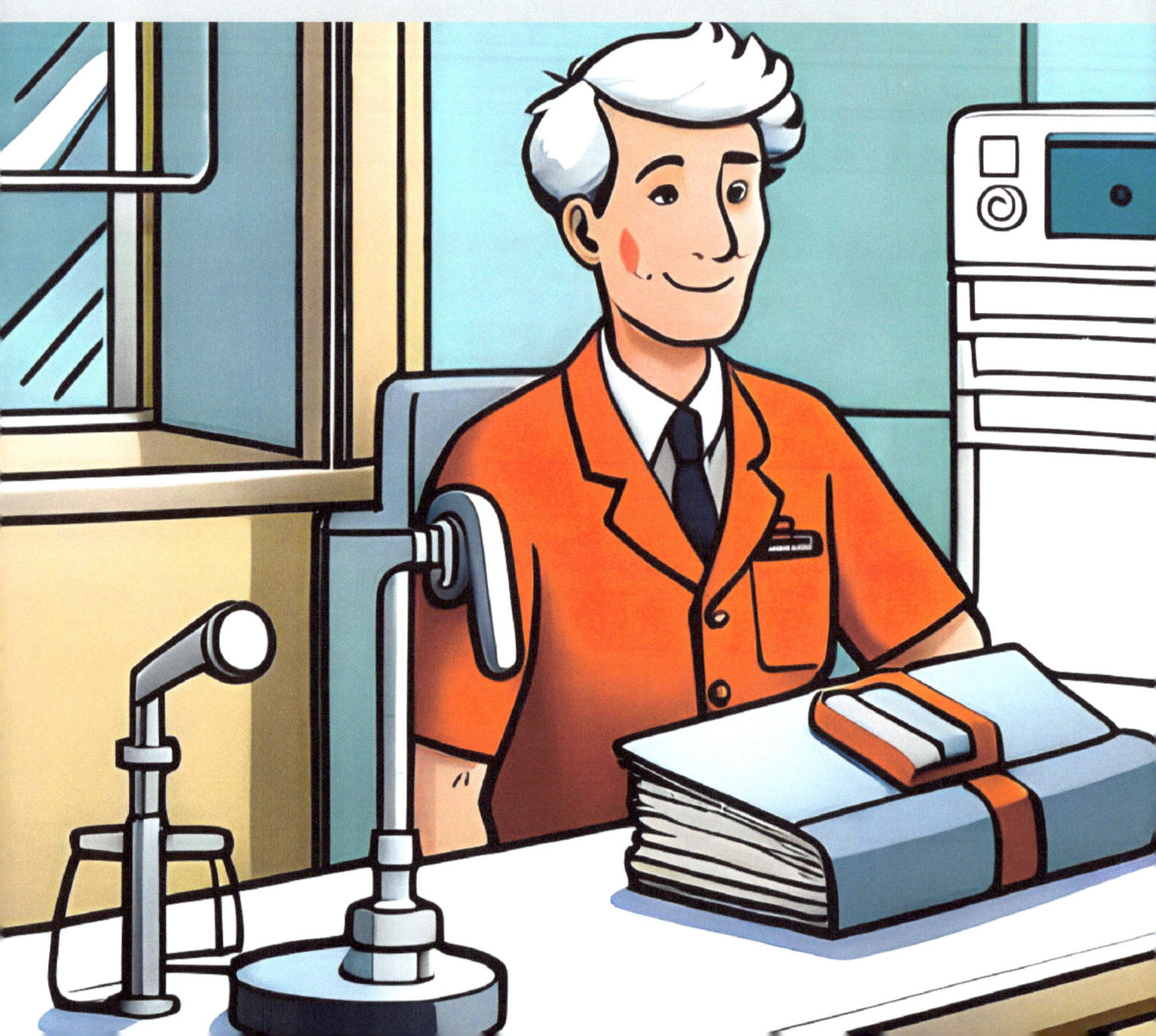

One day, the little veterinarian noticed that their dog Max was not feeling well. Max seemed lethargic and didn't have much of an appetite. Concerned, the little veterinarian decided it was time for a visit to the vet.

The little veterinarian and Max went to the veterinary clinic, where they were greeted by the receptionist. The little veterinarian was amazed by the sight of all the animals in the waiting room. There were cats, dogs, birds, and even a rabbit!

When it was Max's turn to see the vet, the little veterinarian watched as the vet examined Max from head to tail. The vet used different tools, such as a stethoscope, to listen to Max's heart and lungs. The little veterinarian was fascinated by the equipment and asked the vet about how they worked.

The vet patiently explained how each tool was used to examine different parts of an animal's body. The little veterinarian was amazed by how much the vet knew about animals and how they used their knowledge to help them.

After the exam, the vet prescribed some medicine for Max and gave the little veterinarian some advice on how to take care of him. The little veterinarian thanked the vet and left the clinic, feeling inspired to learn more about the profession.

From that day on, the little veterinarian spent more time reading books about veterinary medicine and watching videos about animal care. The little veterinarian was determined to learn as much as they could about animals and how to help them.

The visit to the vet was a turning point for the little veterinarian, and they knew that they were on the path to achieving their dream of becoming a veterinarian.

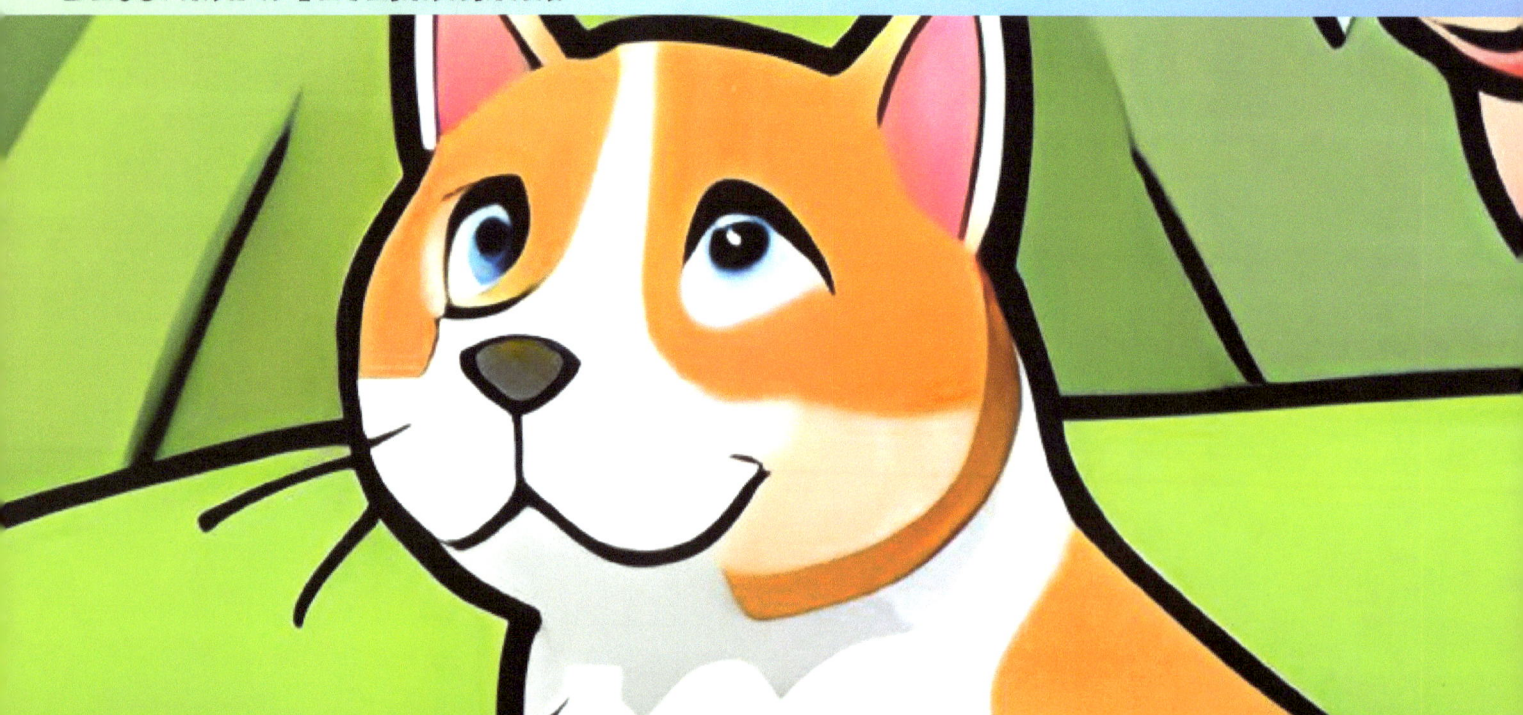

IN A LAND FAR AWAY, WHERE THE TREES GREW TALL,
THERE WAS A LITTLE VILLAGE WHERE MUSIC WAS ALL.
FROM THE SOUND OF THE STREAMS TO THE RUSTLING LEAVES,
THE WORLD WAS A SYMPHONY, AND THE PEOPLE BELIEVED.

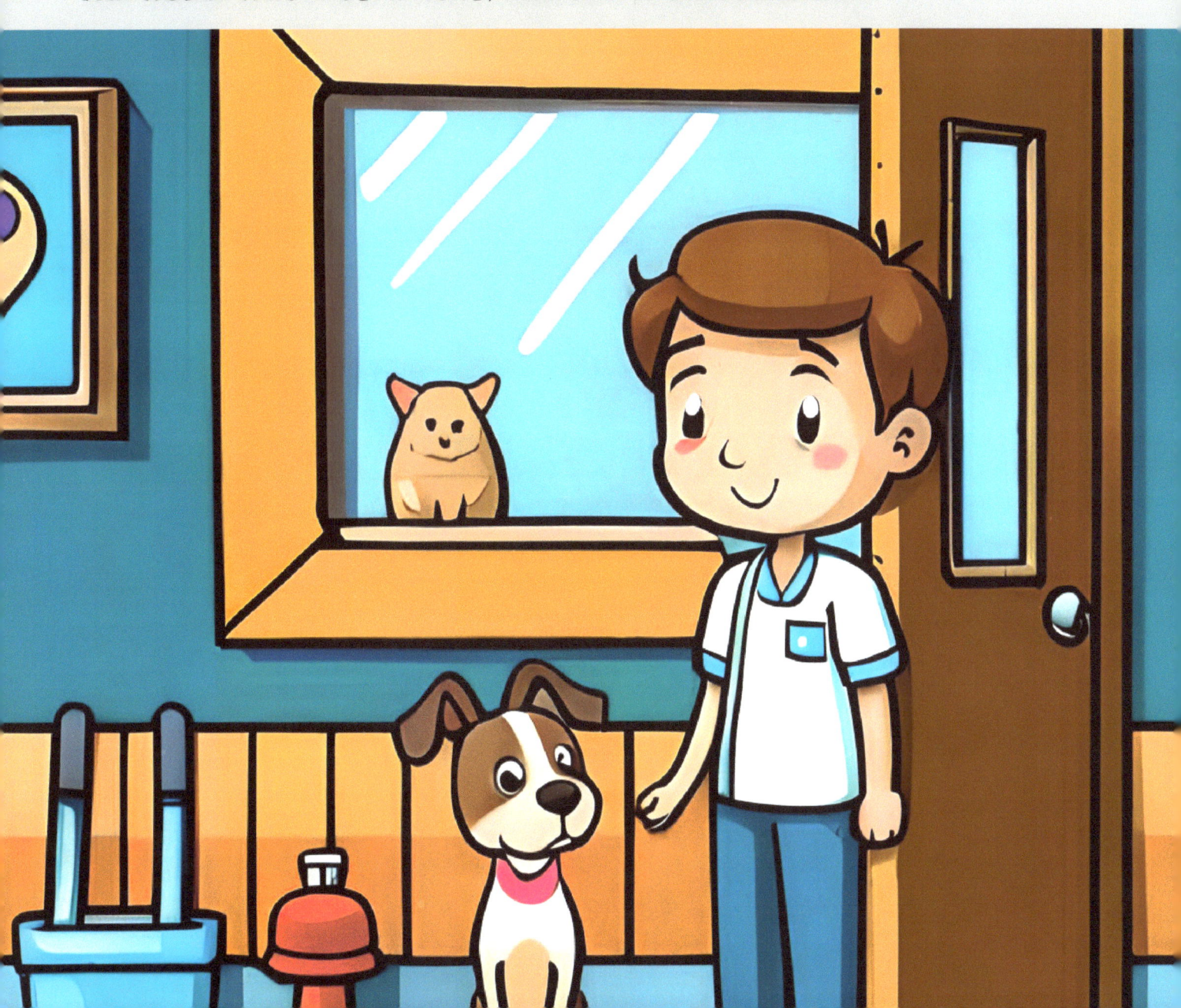

THEY DANCED AND SANG WITH ALL THEIR MIGHT,
FROM MORNING TILL LATE INTO THE NIGHT.
WITH FEET THAT TAPPED AND HANDS THAT CLAPPED,
THEY MADE MUSIC THAT NEVER STOPPED.

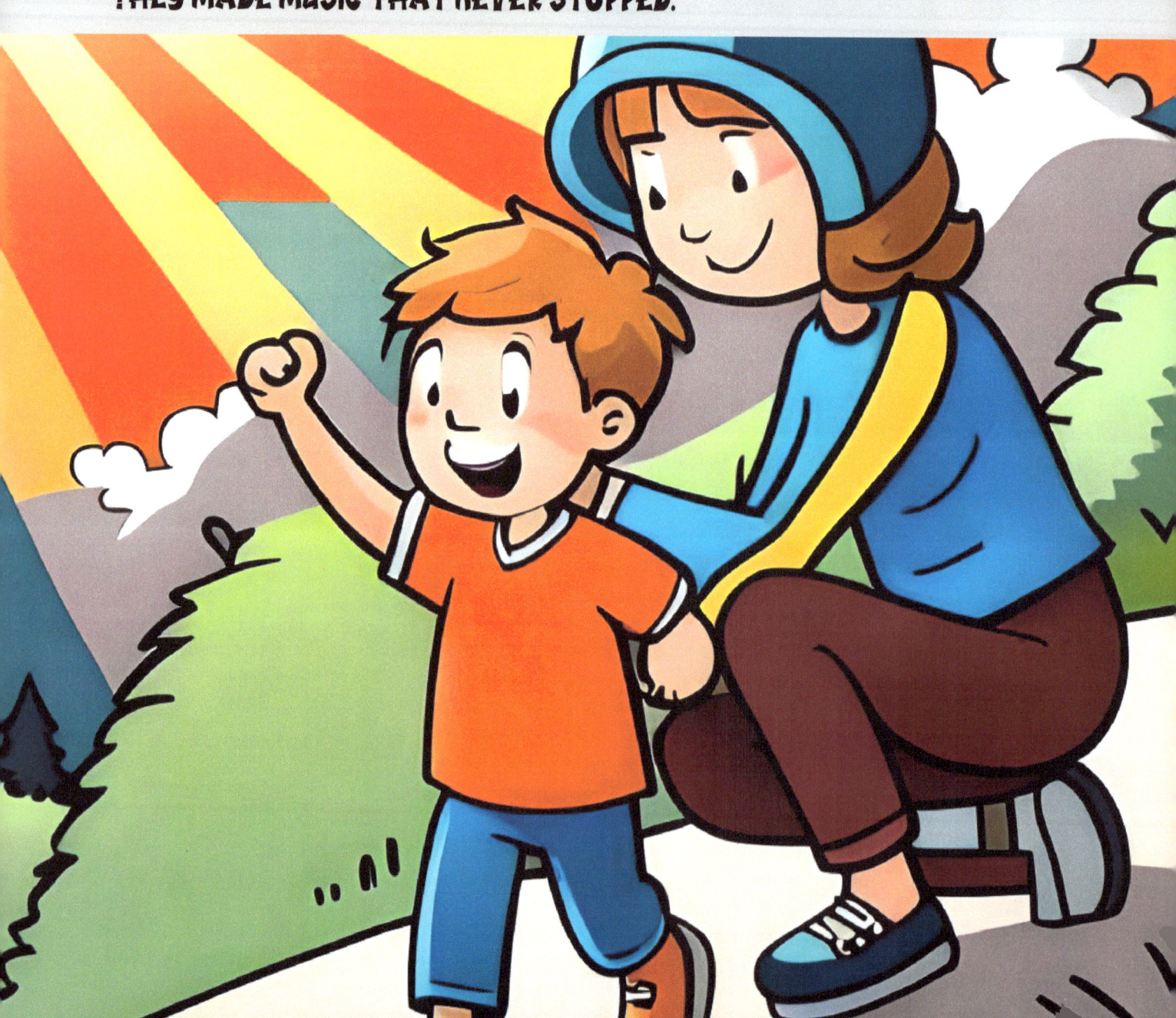

From the village square to the fields of gold,
The rhythm of life was a story told.
With every step and every beat,
The music was their heart and their feet.

They played on flutes, they played on drums,
They played on harps, and lutes, and hummed.
Their voices rose high, with a melody sweet,
And the world around them moved to the beat.

For in this land of rhythm and song,
The people knew where they belonged.
With music in their soul and a beat in their heart,
They lived each day with a joy that never did part.

So if you ever wander to this land so fair,
Listen closely to the music in the air.
Let it fill your heart, and let it guide your way,
For in this land of rhythm, happiness forever will stay.

CHAPTER 3: THE BASICS OF ANIMAL CARE

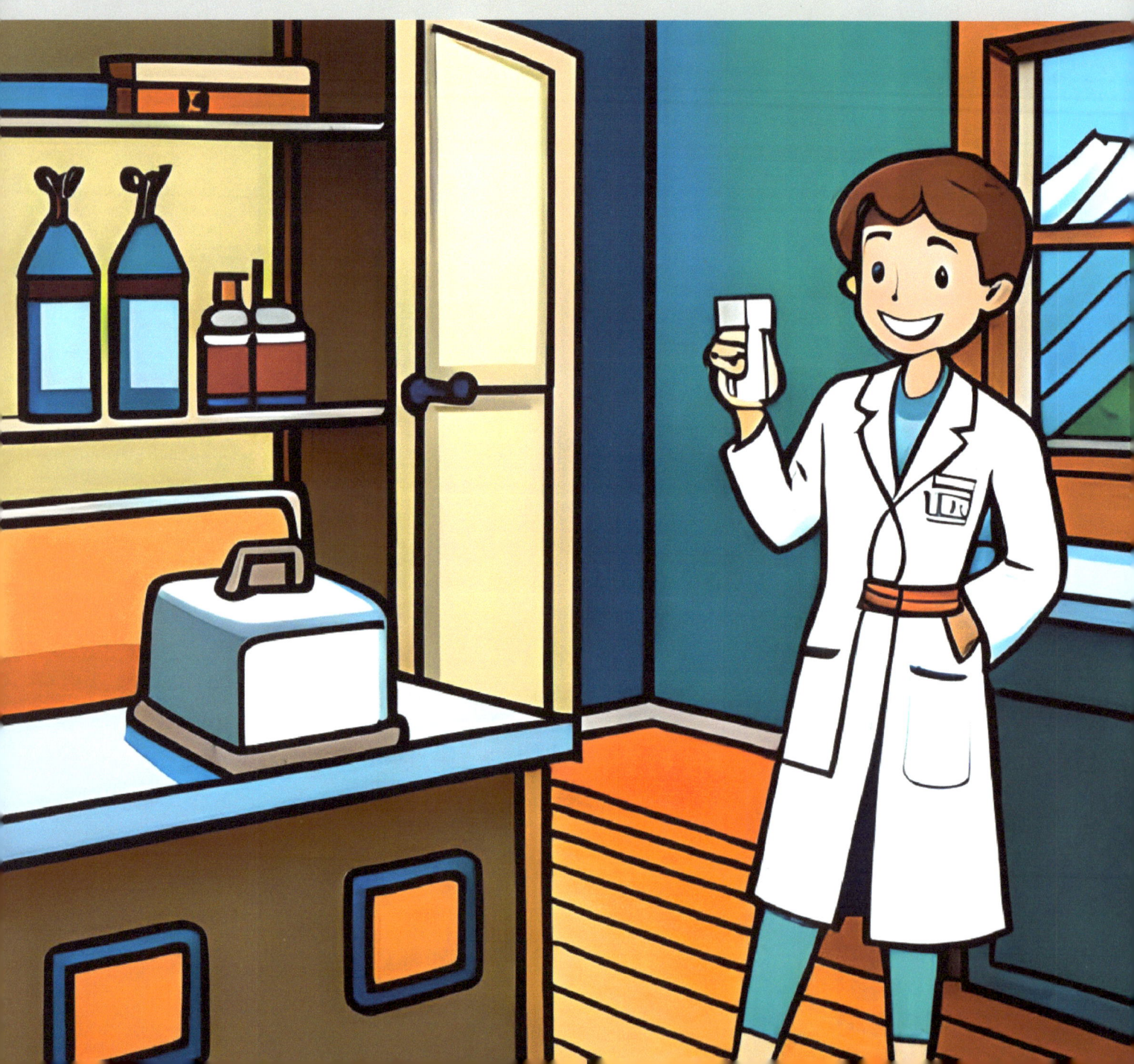

After the visit to the vet, the little veterinarian was even more determined to learn all they could about animal care. They started by researching the basics of pet care, including nutrition, exercise, and hygiene.

The little veterinarian learned that it was important to feed pets a balanced diet that included protein, carbohydrates, and vitamins. They also learned about the dangers of overfeeding and the importance of portion control.

Next, the little veterinarian learned about the importance of exercise for pets. They learned that regular exercise not only keeps pets physically healthy but also mentally stimulated. The little veterinarian started taking Max on longer walks and playing more games with him.

The little veterinarian also learned about the importance of hygiene in pet care. They learned about the proper way to bathe and groom pets, as well as how to clean their teeth and ears. They even practiced brushing Max's teeth and cleaning his ears.

As the little veterinarian continued to learn about animal care, they also learned how to identify common health problems in pets. They learned how to check for fleas and ticks and how to spot signs of ear infections.

THE LITTLE VETERINARIAN WAS AMAZED BY HOW MUCH THERE WAS TO LEARN ABOUT TAKING CARE OF ANIMALS. THEY FELT EMPOWERED BY THE KNOWLEDGE THEY HAD GAINED AND KNEW THAT THEY COULD USE IT TO HELP MAX AND OTHER PETS IN THEIR COMMUNITY.

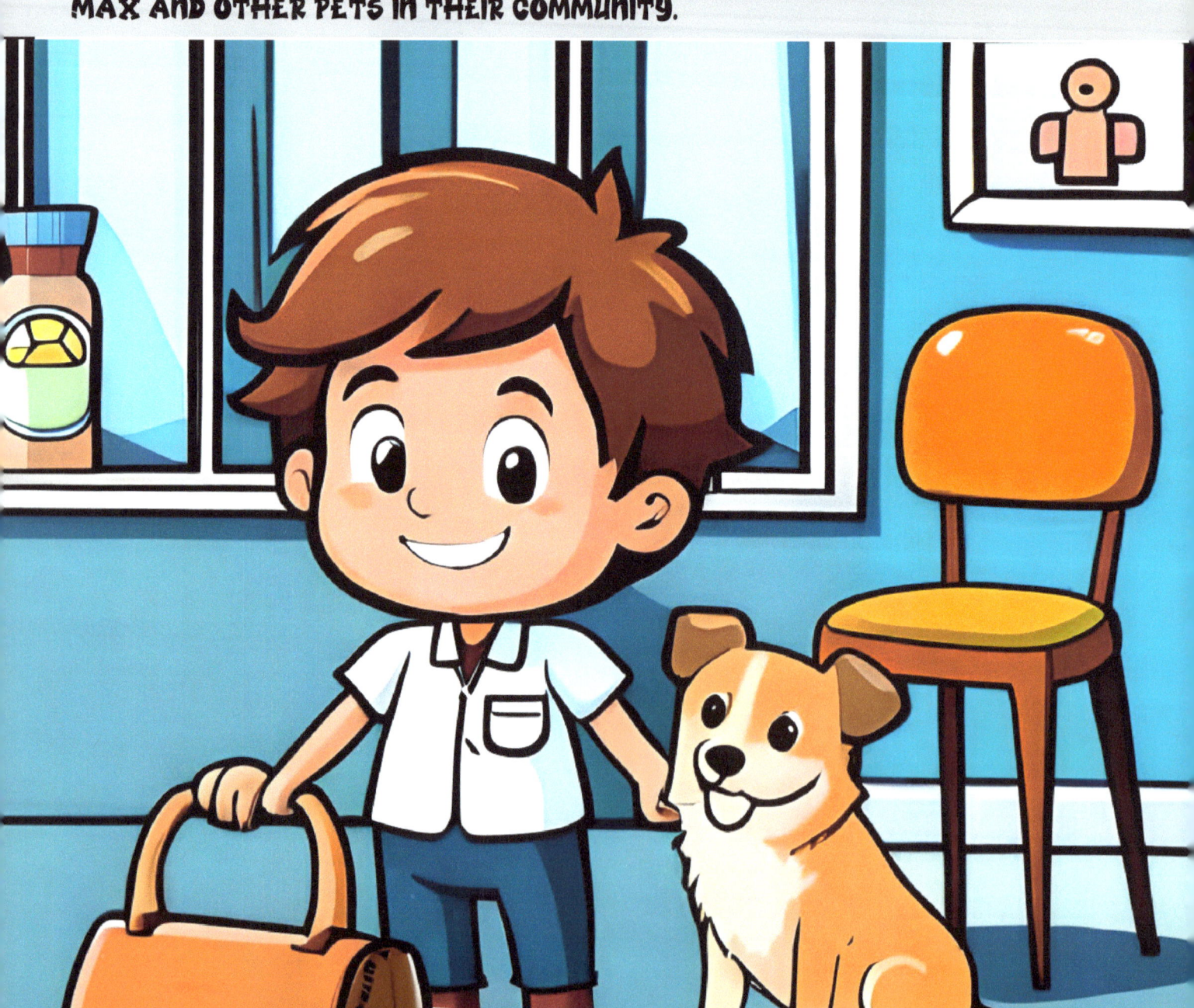

From that day on, the little veterinarian continued to learn and grow their knowledge about animal care. They knew that they still had a lot to learn, but they were excited about the journey ahead.

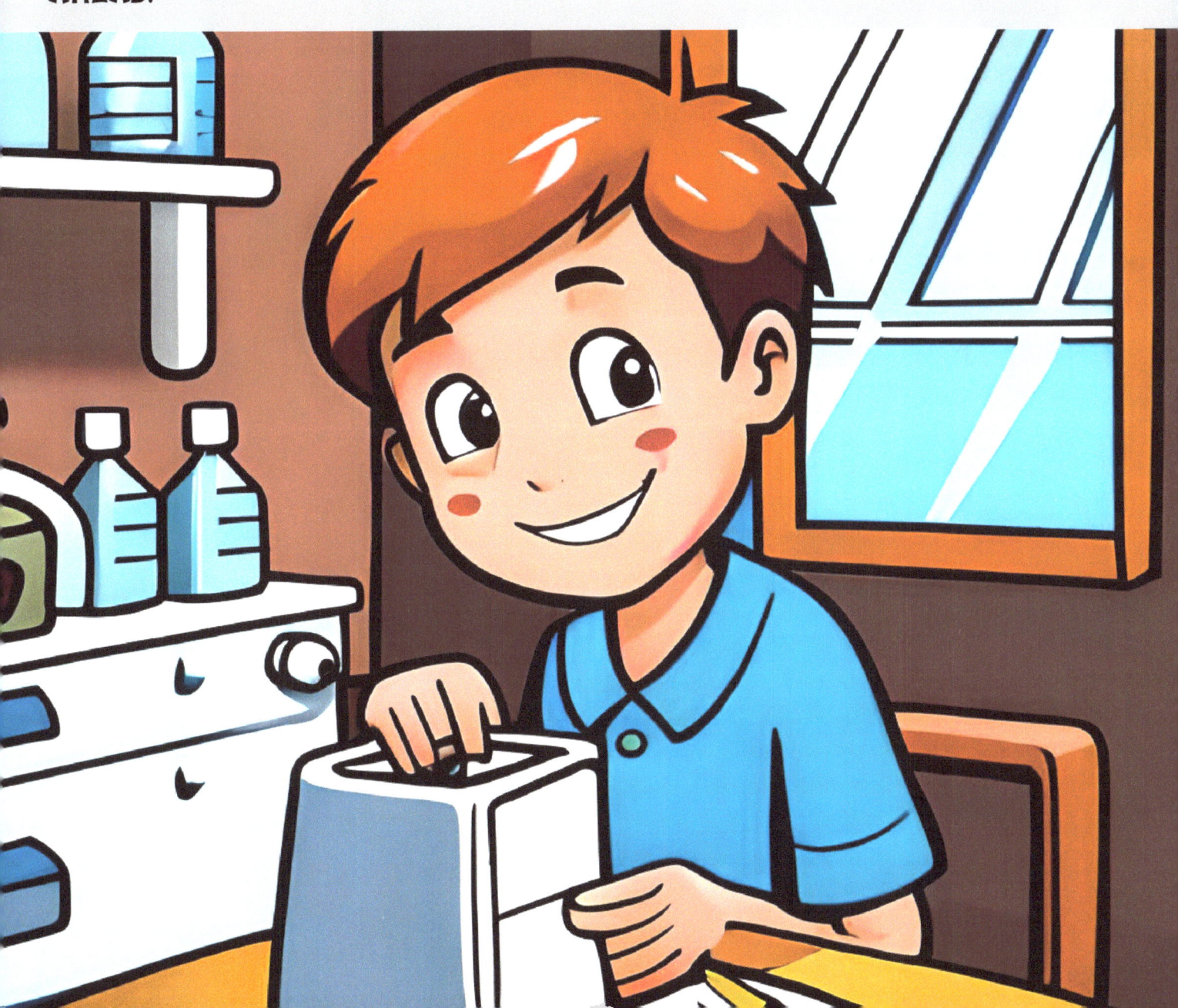

IN A LAND OF ENDLESS SKIES AND ROLLING HILLS,
THERE LIVED A GIRL WHO LOVED TO PLAY AND SING.
SHE DANCED THROUGH FIELDS AND OVER HILLS,
AND EVERY STEP WAS LIKE A JOYFUL THING.

SHE SANG OF LOVE AND OF THE STARS ABOVE,
AND EVERY NOTE WAS LIKE A BEAM OF LIGHT.
SHE PLAYED HER GUITAR AND STRUMMED WITH LOVE,
AND EVERYTHING AROUND HER FELT JUST RIGHT.

HER MUSIC FILLED THE AIR AND TOUCHED THE HEARTS,
OF ALL WHO HEARD HER SWEET AND JOYFUL SOUND.
FROM THE BIRDS IN THE TREES TO THE BEES IN THE HIVE,
THE WORLD AROUND HER DANCED AND TWIRLED AROUND.

FOR MUSIC WAS HER GIFT, HER JOY, HER LIGHT,
AND EVERY NOTE WAS LIKE A BURST OF PURE DELIGHT.
AND AS SHE PLAYED AND SANG WITH ALL HER MIGHT,
THE WORLD AROUND HER FELT SO PURE AND BRIGHT.

SO IF YOU EVER WANDER THROUGH THIS LAND SO GRAND,
LISTEN CLOSELY TO THE GIRL WHO SINGS AND PLAYS.
LET HER MUSIC GUIDE YOU TO A WONDROUS PLACE,
WHERE JOY AND LOVE FILL EVERY SINGLE DAY.

CHAPTER 4: ANATOMY AND PHYSIOLOGY

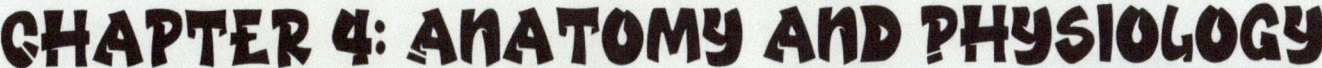

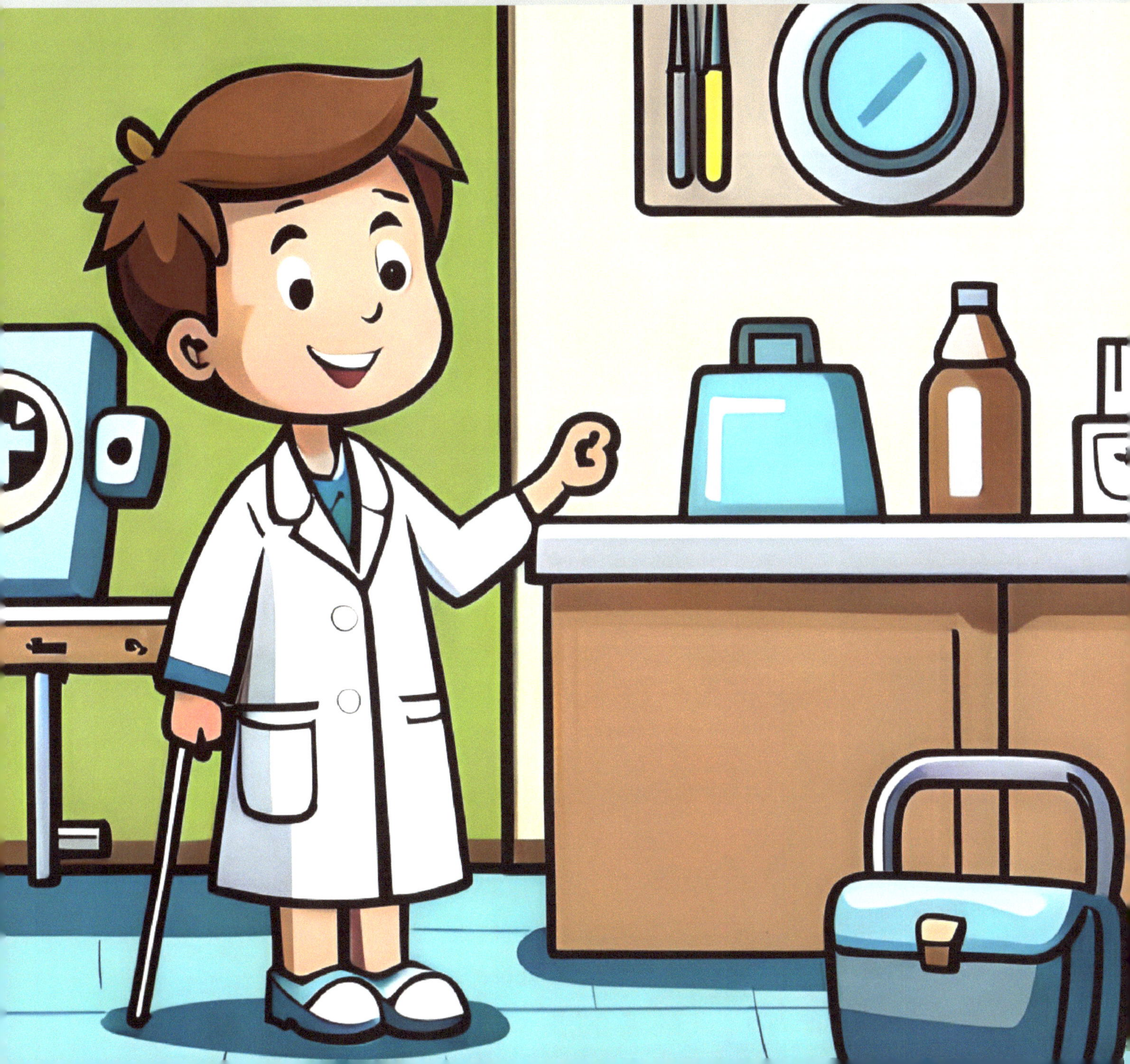

The little veterinarian was fascinated by the intricacies of the animal body. They started to study the different body systems, including the respiratory, circulatory, and digestive systems.

The little veterinarian learned that the respiratory system is responsible for breathing and supplying oxygen to the body. They learned about common respiratory illnesses, like coughing and sneezing, and how to treat them with medication.

Next, the little veterinarian studied the circulatory system, which is responsible for transporting blood and nutrients throughout the body. They learned about the importance of regular check-ups to detect any heart problems early and how to treat common illnesses like heartworm.

Finally, the little veterinarian learned about the digestive system, which is responsible for breaking down food and absorbing nutrients. They learned about common digestive problems like diarrhea and vomiting and how to treat them with dietary changes and medication.

The little veterinarian was amazed by the complexity of the animal body and how each system worked together to keep animals healthy. They knew that with this knowledge, they could help keep their own pet, Max, healthy and potentially save the lives of other animals in need.

As the little veterinarian continued their studies, they realized that becoming a veterinarian would take years of hard work and dedication. But they were determined to continue learning and growing their knowledge until they could make a real difference in the lives of animals.

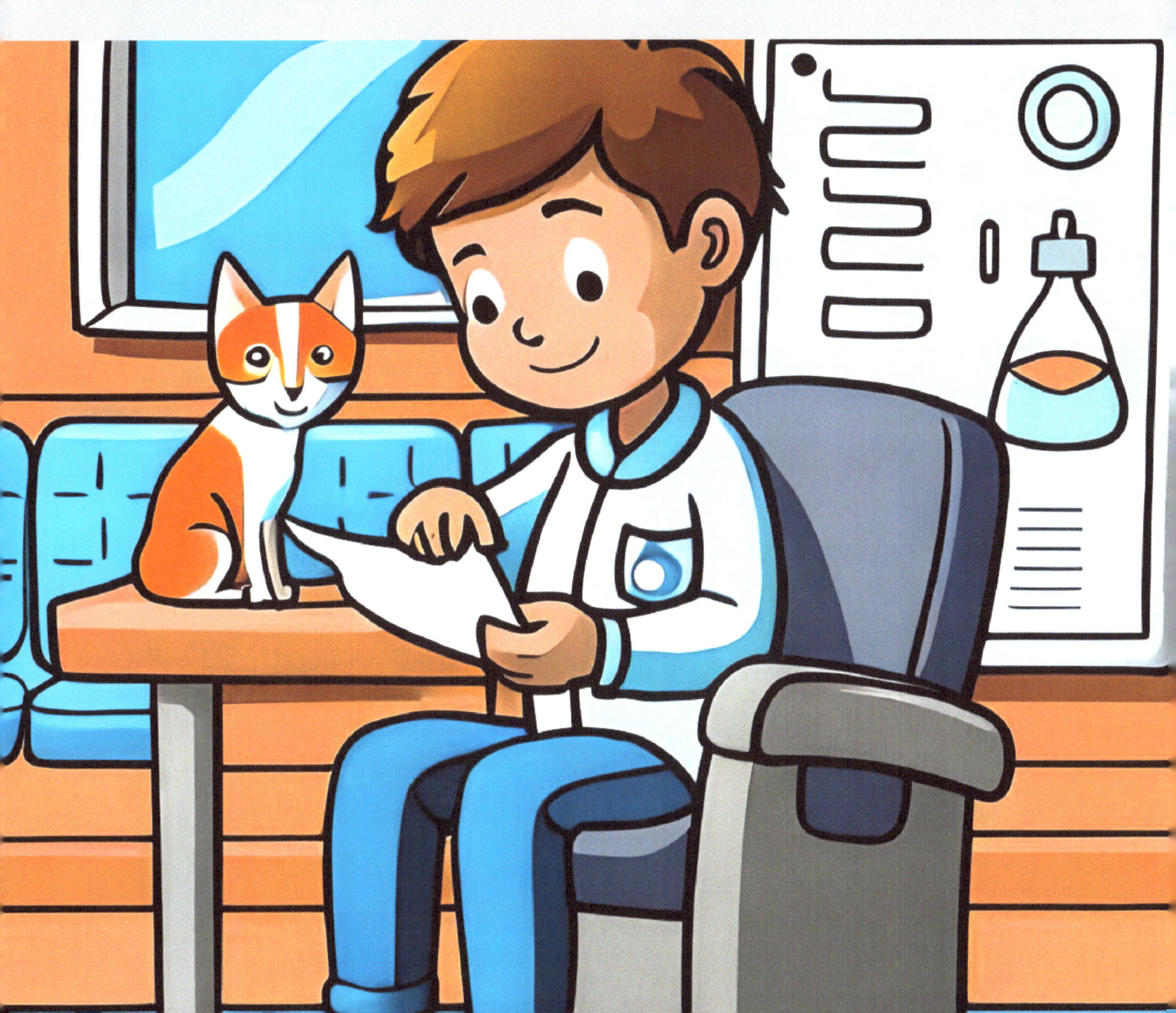

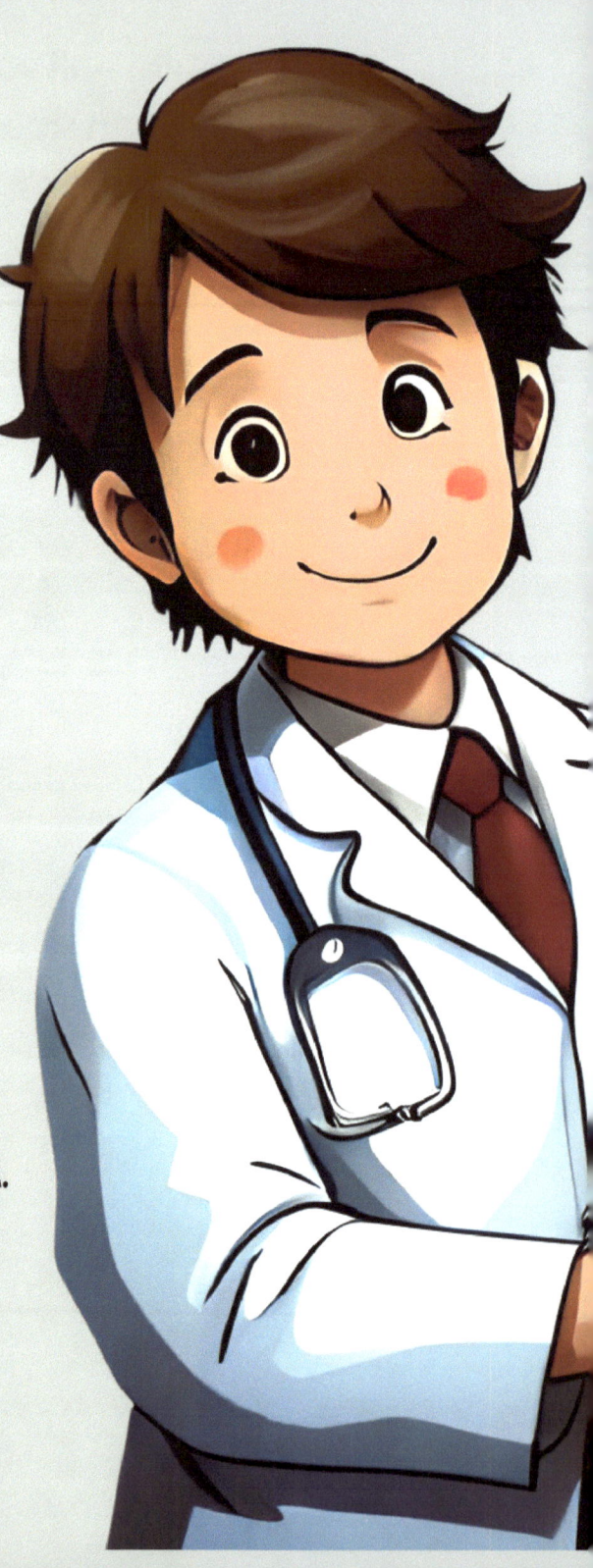

The sun sets low over the rolling hills,
As the moon and stars begin to rise.
The world around is peaceful and still,
As a little bird sings a lullaby.

The melody is soft, gentle and sweet,
As the bird sings to the world below.
Its voice a soothing, comforting treat,
That washes over all that it knows.

The night sky is filled with twinkling light,
As the bird sings its song of the night.
Its voice a beacon in the dark of the night,
Guiding all to a place of calm and delight.

As the bird sings, the world is at peace,
With all the troubles of the day now ceased.
The melody lingers, a sweet release,
From the worries and cares that never cease.

So listen close to the bird's sweet song,
And let its music carry you along.
To a world of peace, where nothing's wrong,
And the melody of life is forever strong.

CHAPTER 5: EMERGENCY MEDICINE

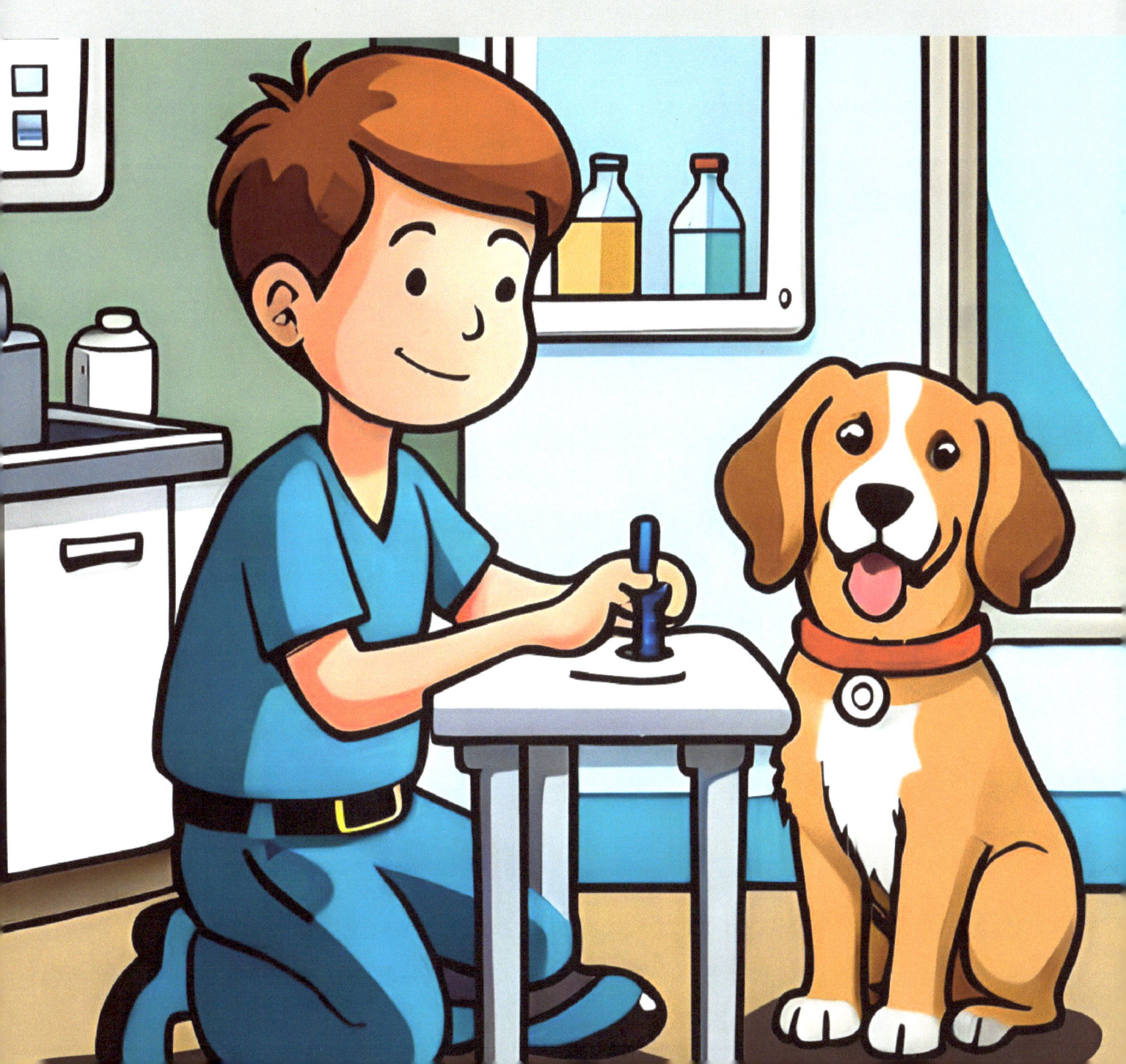

The little veterinarian knew that emergencies can happen at any time, and it's important to be prepared. They started to study first aid and emergency care for pets.

The little veterinarian learned about CPR and how to perform it on both dogs and cats. They also learned how to handle emergencies like choking, bleeding, and seizures.

They practiced different techniques for helping animals who are choking, like the Heimlich maneuver, and how to stop bleeding by applying pressure to the wound.

The little veterinarian also learned about common signs of seizures in pets, like trembling, loss of consciousness, and muscle spasms. They learned how to keep the animal safe during a seizure and when to seek veterinary care.

As the little veterinarian practiced these emergency techniques, they realized how important it was to be prepared. They knew that in a real emergency, they would need to act quickly and calmly to help the animal in need.

The little veterinarian felt empowered by their knowledge and knew that they could make a real difference in the lives of animals. They felt confident in their ability to help their own pet, Max, and potentially save the lives of other animals in an emergency.

As they continued their studies, the little veterinarian knew that they were one step closer to achieving their dream of becoming a veterinarian and helping animals in need.

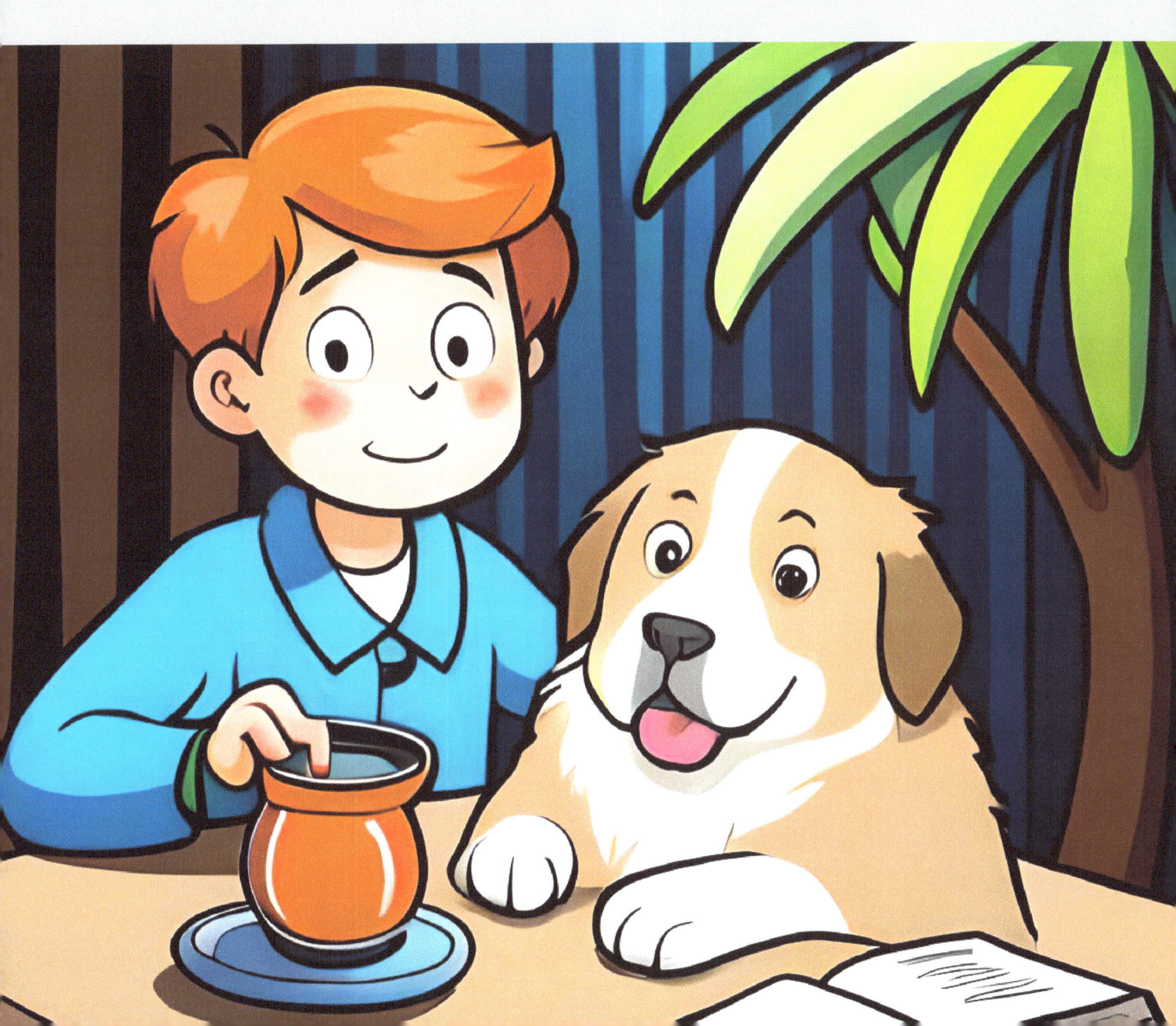

In the early morning light,
As the sun begins to rise,
The world awakens to a brand new day,
Filled with hope and surprise.

The birds sing out in joyful song,
Their melodies pure and bright,
As they welcome in the new day,
With a symphony of light.

The flowers open up their petals,
Revealing their beauty to the world,
Their colors shining bright and bold,
Like banners being unfurled.

The trees sway gently in the breeze,
Their branches reaching to the sky,
As they stand tall and strong,
Watching the world go by.

And in the midst of this new day,
A little veterinarian stands proud,
With a heart full of hope and passion,
And a dream that's not allowed.

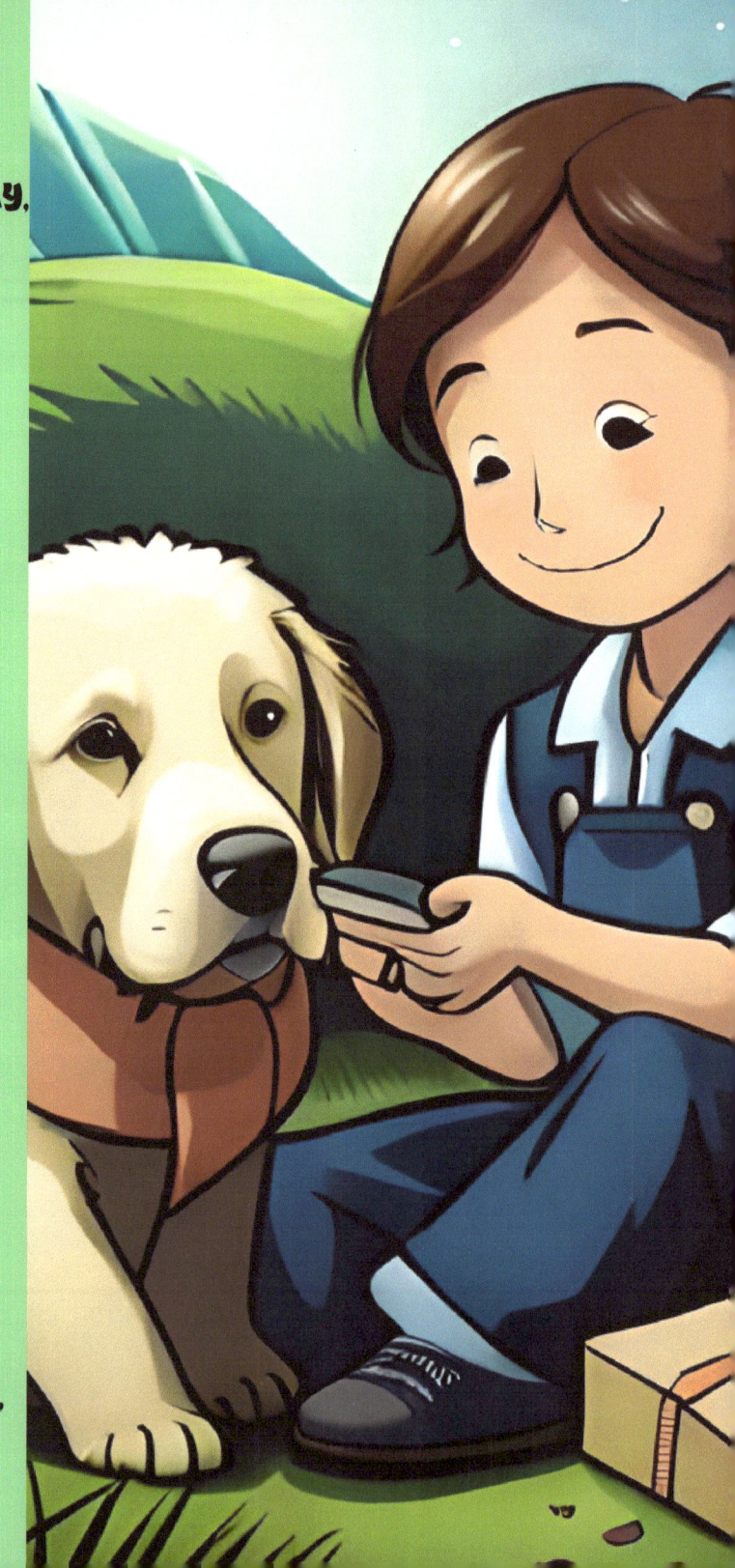

For this little veterinarian knows,
that the world can be a better place,
with a little love and compassion,
and a smile on every face.

So they study hard and work each day,
with a goal that's clear in sight,
to help animals in need,
and to make the world a little more bright.

For in this brand new day,
filled with hope and surprise,
the little veterinarian knows,
that anything is possible, if they just try.

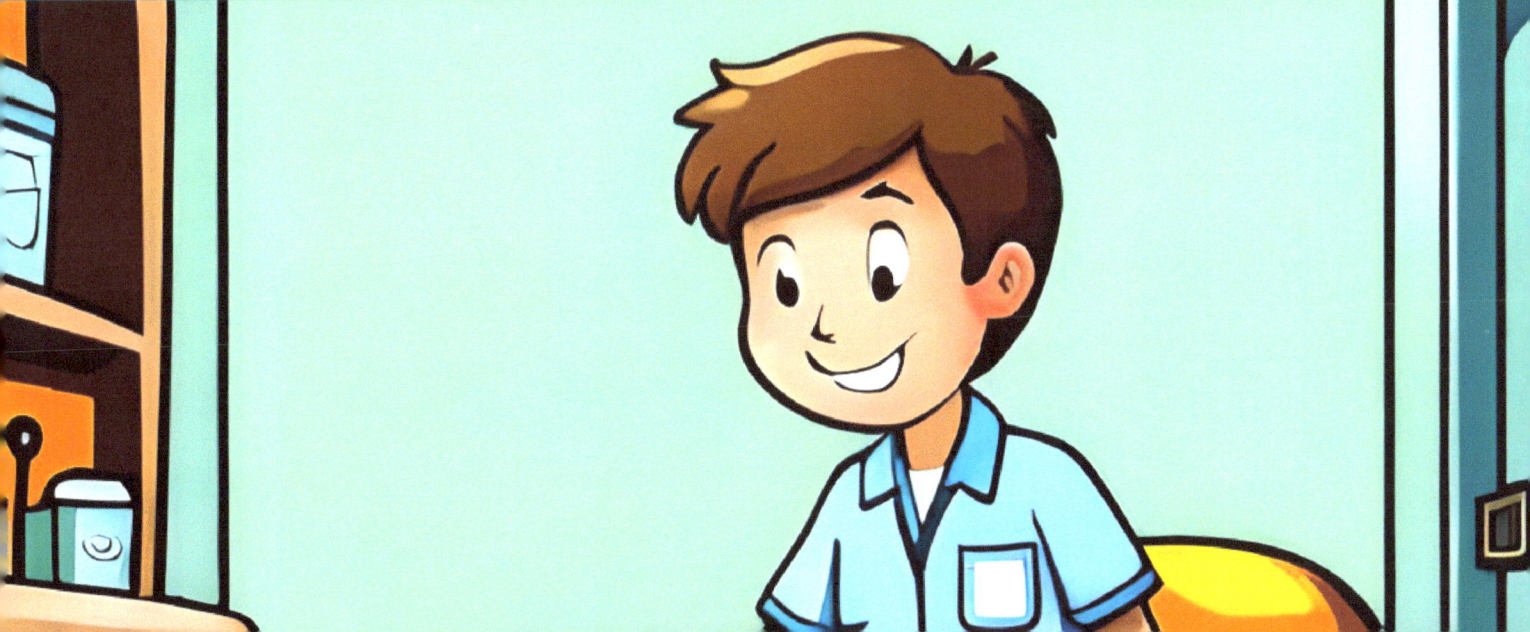

CHAPTER 6: SURGERY AND REHABILITATION

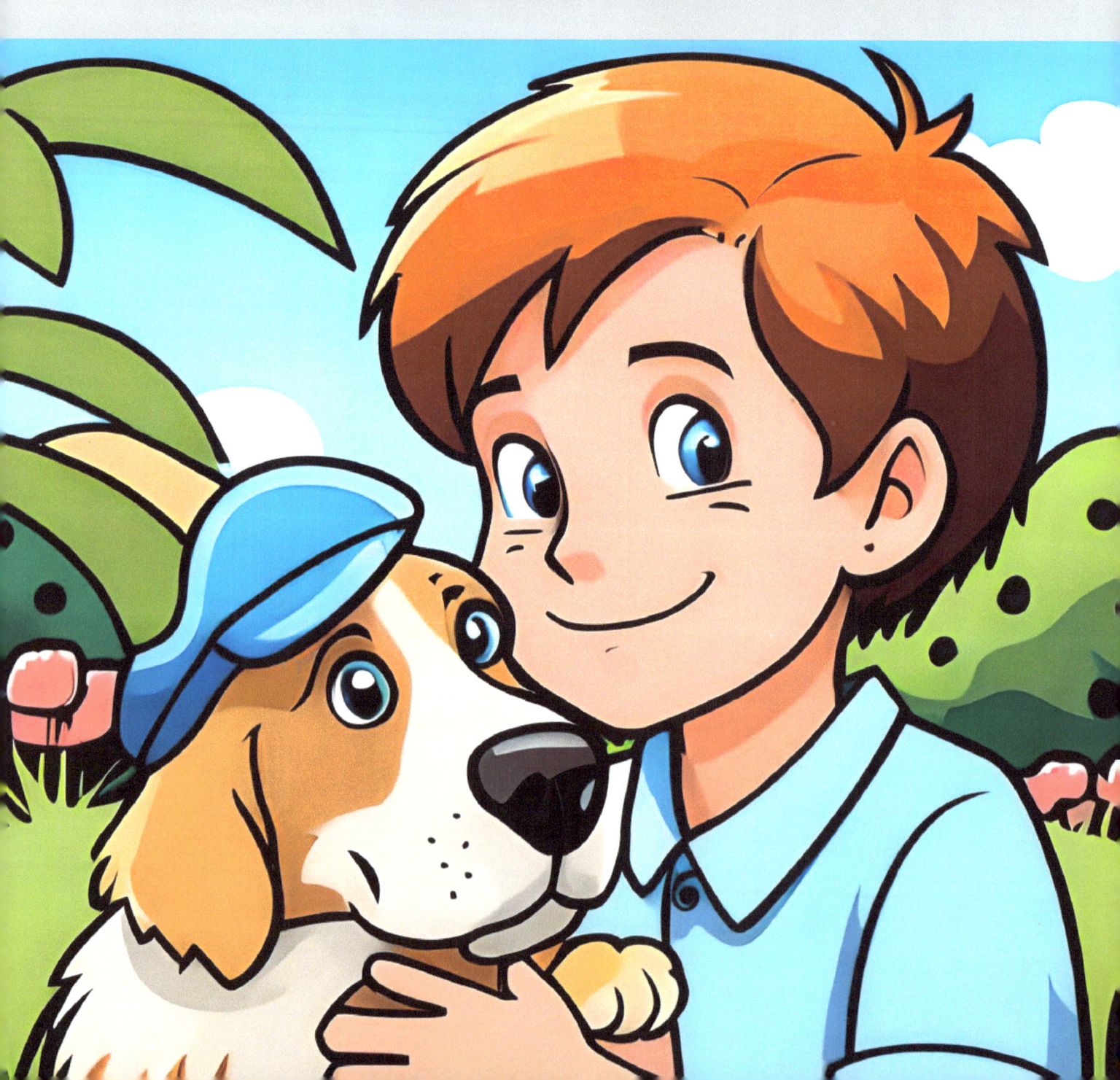

The little veterinarian continued to study and learn about all aspects of animal health and care. One day, they had the opportunity to observe a surgery at a veterinary clinic.

As they watched the veterinarian carefully perform the surgery, the little veterinarian learned about the different types of surgeries that animals may need. They saw how a spaying or neutering surgery was performed, which helps control the animal population and reduces the risk of certain diseases.

They also saw how tumors could be removed and how broken bones could be repaired. The little veterinarian was fascinated by the complexity of the surgeries and how the veterinarian used different tools and techniques to ensure the animal's safety and well-being.

After the surgery, the little veterinarian learned about the importance of rehabilitation and physical therapy for animals recovering from surgery or injuries. They saw how exercises and therapies could help improve an animal's strength, flexibility, and mobility.

The little veterinarian also learned about the importance of monitoring the animal's progress and adjusting the therapy accordingly. They saw how each animal's needs were unique and how important it was to provide individualized care.

As they left the clinic, the little veterinarian felt grateful for the opportunity to learn about surgeries and rehabilitation. He knew that these skills would be important for their future as a veterinarian, and he felt inspired to continue his studies and help animals in need.

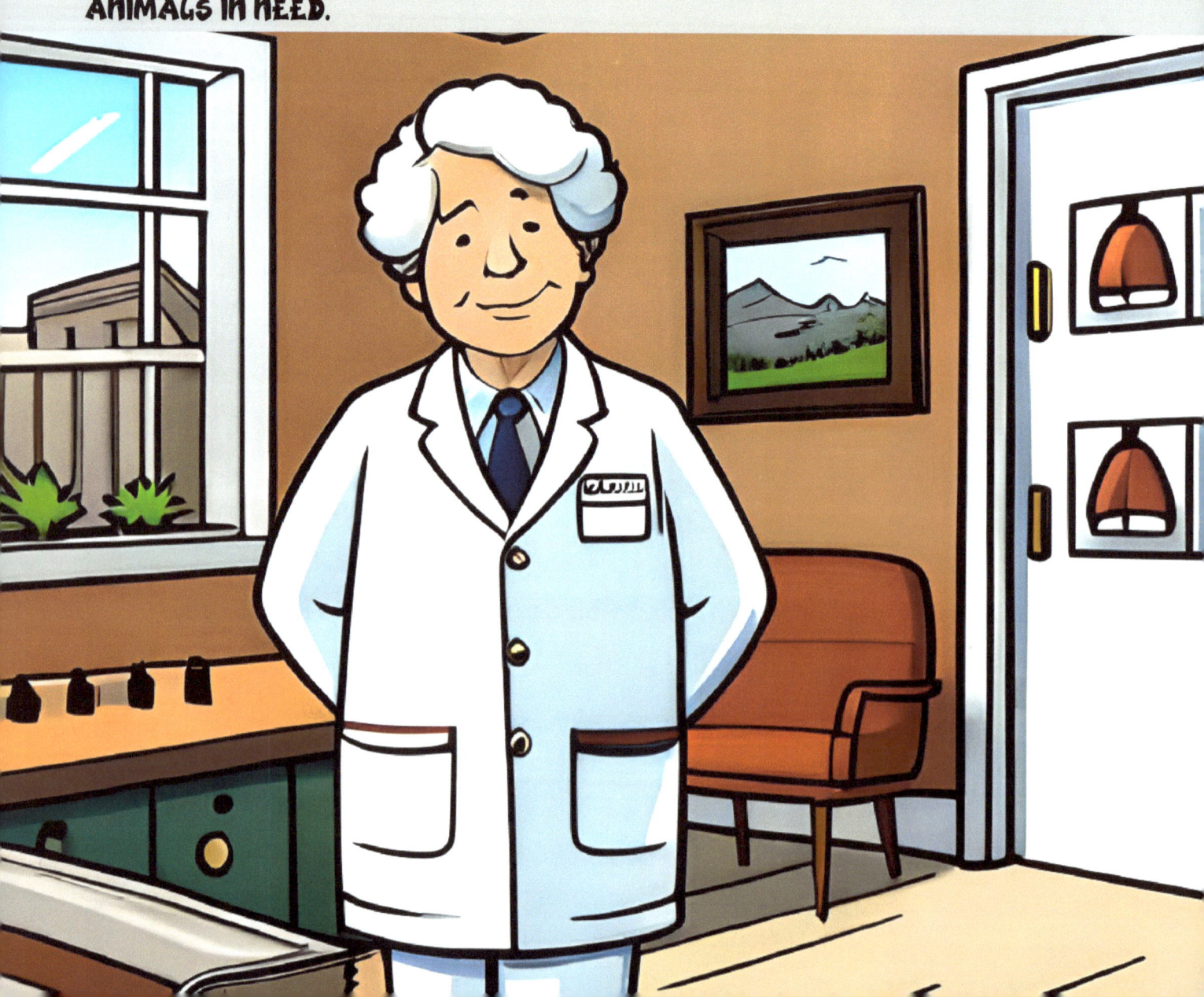

In the bright and bustling clinic,
The little veterinarian did roam,
Observing surgeries with precision,
And learning as they roamed.

They saw the spaying and neutering,
A crucial step in pet health care,
Reducing the risk of diseases,
And preventing unwanted litters there.

They witnessed the tumor removal,
A delicate procedure indeed,
Removing growths to save lives,
A critical task to succeed.

And as they watched the bone repair,
Their eyes opened wide,
Seeing how the vet mended breaks,
And set things back to the animal's side.

The little veterinarian also learned,
About rehabilitation and therapy,
Exercises to improve strength,
And ensure animals' mobility.

FOR EVERY ANIMAL WAS UNIQUE,
WITH ITS OWN SET OF NEEDS,
AND WITH CAREFUL OBSERVATION,
THE LITTLE VETERINARIAN COULD SUCCEED.

WITH A HEART FULL OF PASSION,
AND KNOWLEDGE DEEP AND TRUE,
THE LITTLE VETERINARIAN KNEW,
THAT ANYTHING THEY WANTED TO DO, THEY COULD PURSUE.

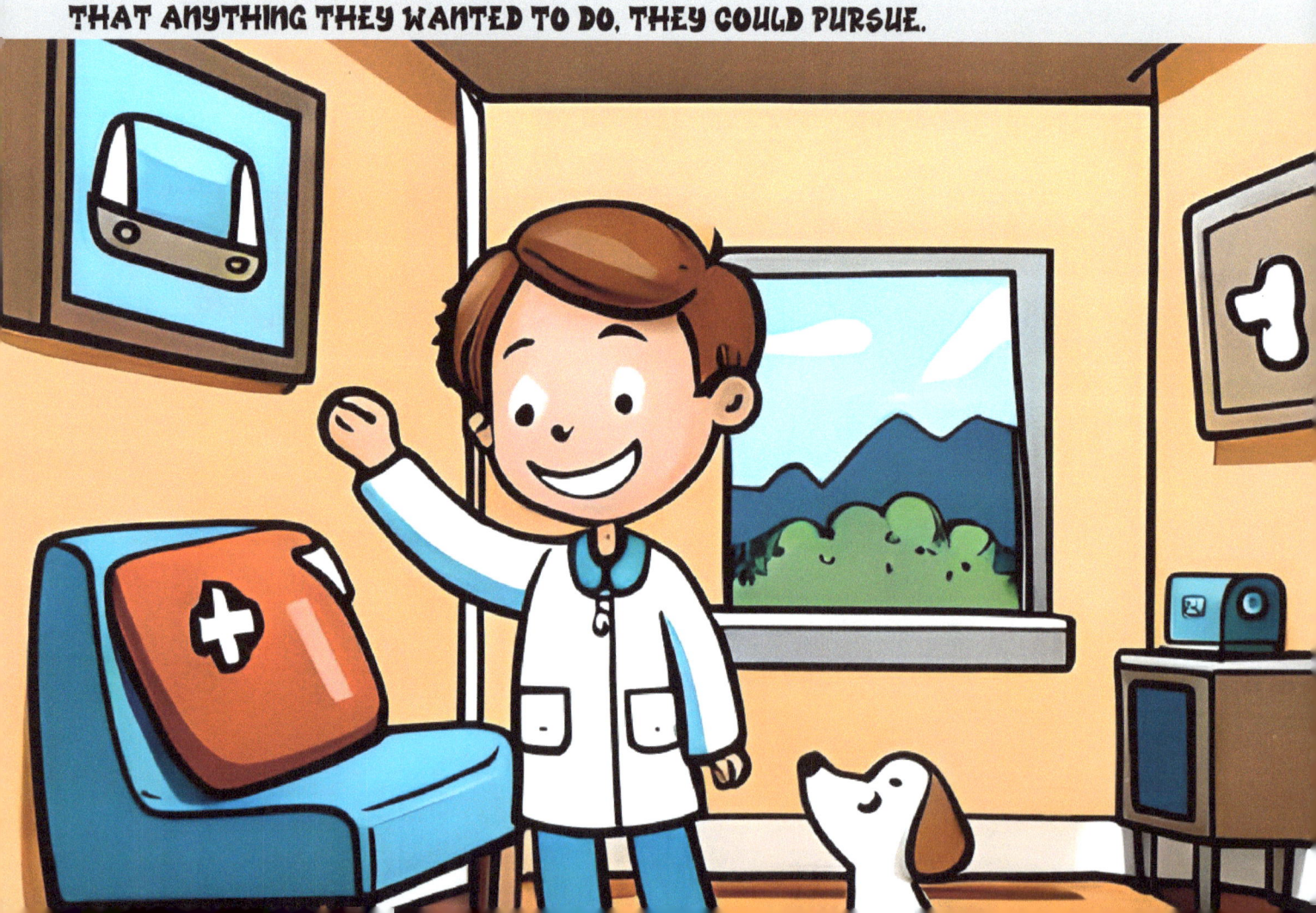

CHAPTER 7: SPECIALIZATIONS IN VETERINARY MEDICINE

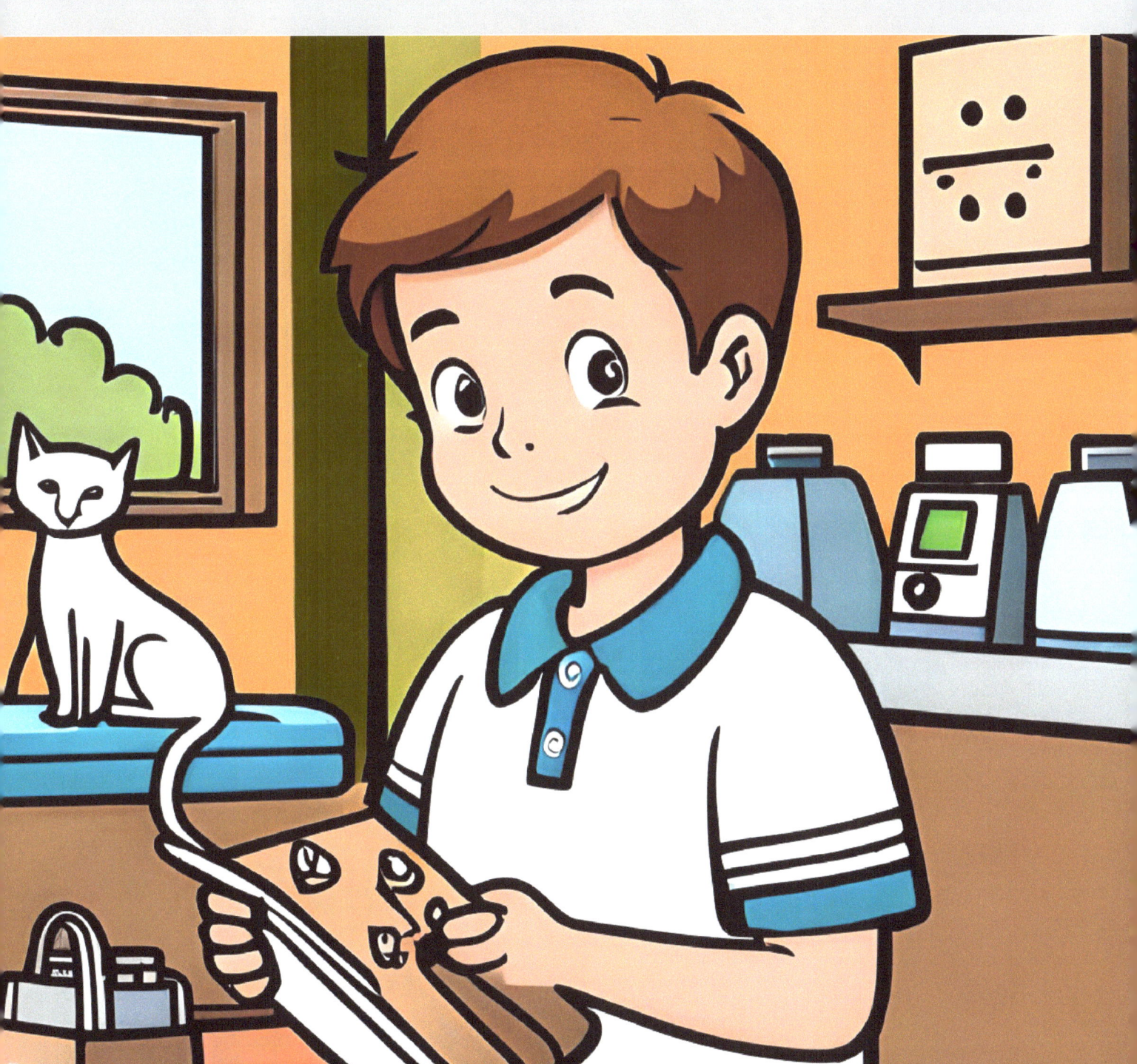

The little veterinarian continued to explore the world of veterinary medicine and discovered that there were many different specializations within the profession. They learned that veterinarians could work with all types of animals, from small pets like cats and dogs to exotic animals like snakes, birds, and even zoo animals.

The little veterinarian was especially interested in the different roles of vet techs, veterinary assistants, and animal behaviorists. They learned that vet techs and assistants played a crucial role in helping veterinarians with exams, surgeries, and treatments, and that animal behaviorists could help animals with behavioral issues like anxiety, aggression, or phobias.

The little veterinarian also learned about the unique challenges and rewards of working with different types of animals. They discovered that marine mammal veterinarians helped care for dolphins, whales, and seals, and that wildlife veterinarians worked to preserve endangered species and rehabilitate injured animals back into the wild.

The little veterinarian was excited to learn about all the different possibilities within the veterinary profession. They knew that they would have to work hard to gain the skills and knowledge needed for their chosen specialty, but they felt inspired by the many ways they could help animals and make a difference in the world.

In the world of veterinary medicine,
The little veterinarian learned,
Of the many specializations,
And the roles that each discerned.

There were those who worked with exotics,
From snakes to birds and more,
And those who worked with marine mammals,
Like dolphins and seals on the shore.

The little veterinarian discovered,
That each animal had unique needs,
And that working with them was challenging,
But fulfilling indeed.

They learned of vet techs and assistants,
And the vital role they play,
In exams, surgeries, and treatments,
To help animals every day.

And animal behaviorists were a part,
Of this diverse veterinary field,
Helping animals with behavioral issues,
So their quality of life could be healed.

THE LITTLE VETERINARIAN WAS INSPIRED,
BY THE MANY WAYS THEY COULD MAKE A CHANGE,
TO HELP ANIMALS AND THEIR OWNERS,
IN A PROFESSION THAT'S TRULY AMAZING AND STRANGE.

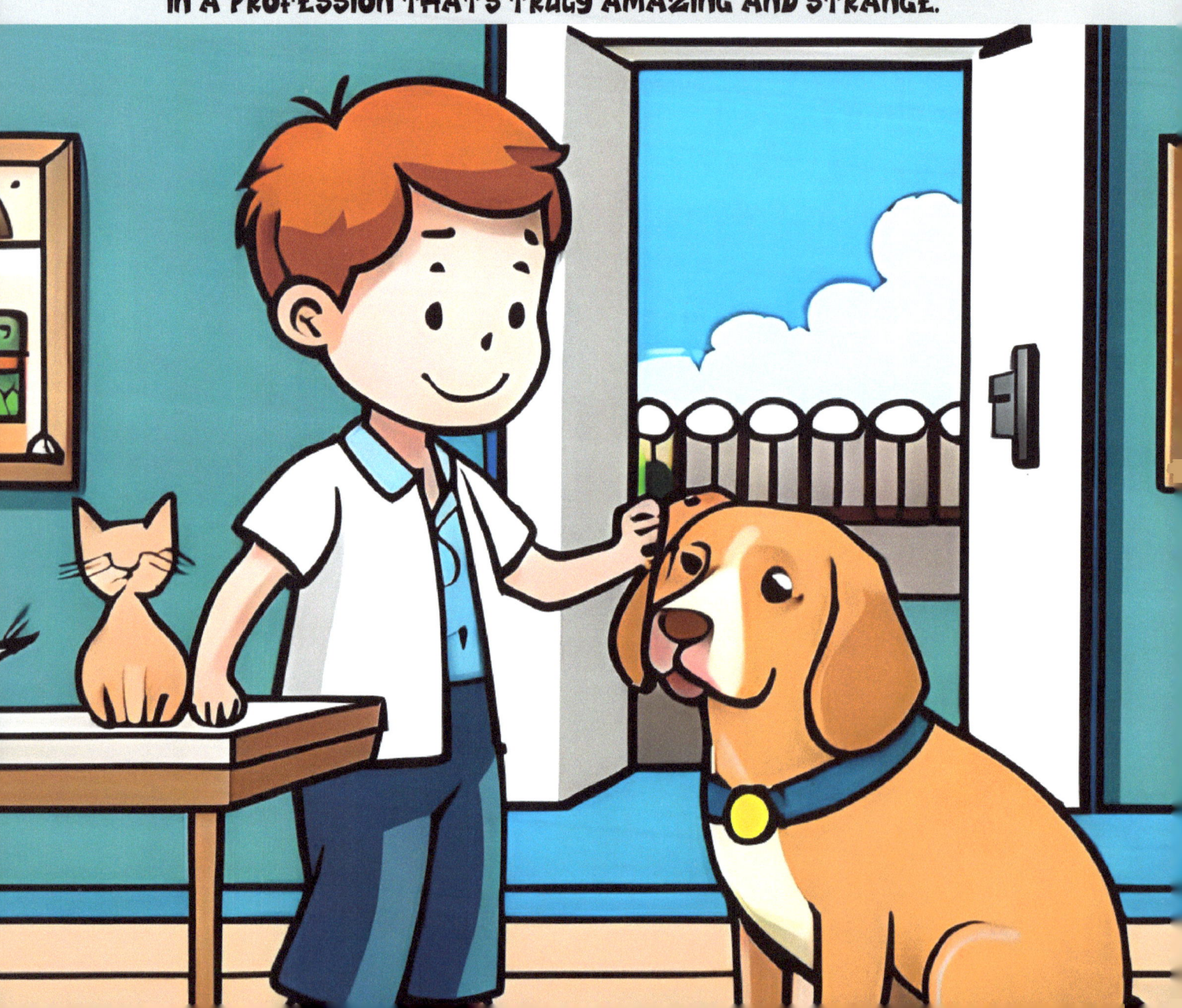

CHAPTER 8: BECOMING A VETERINARIAN

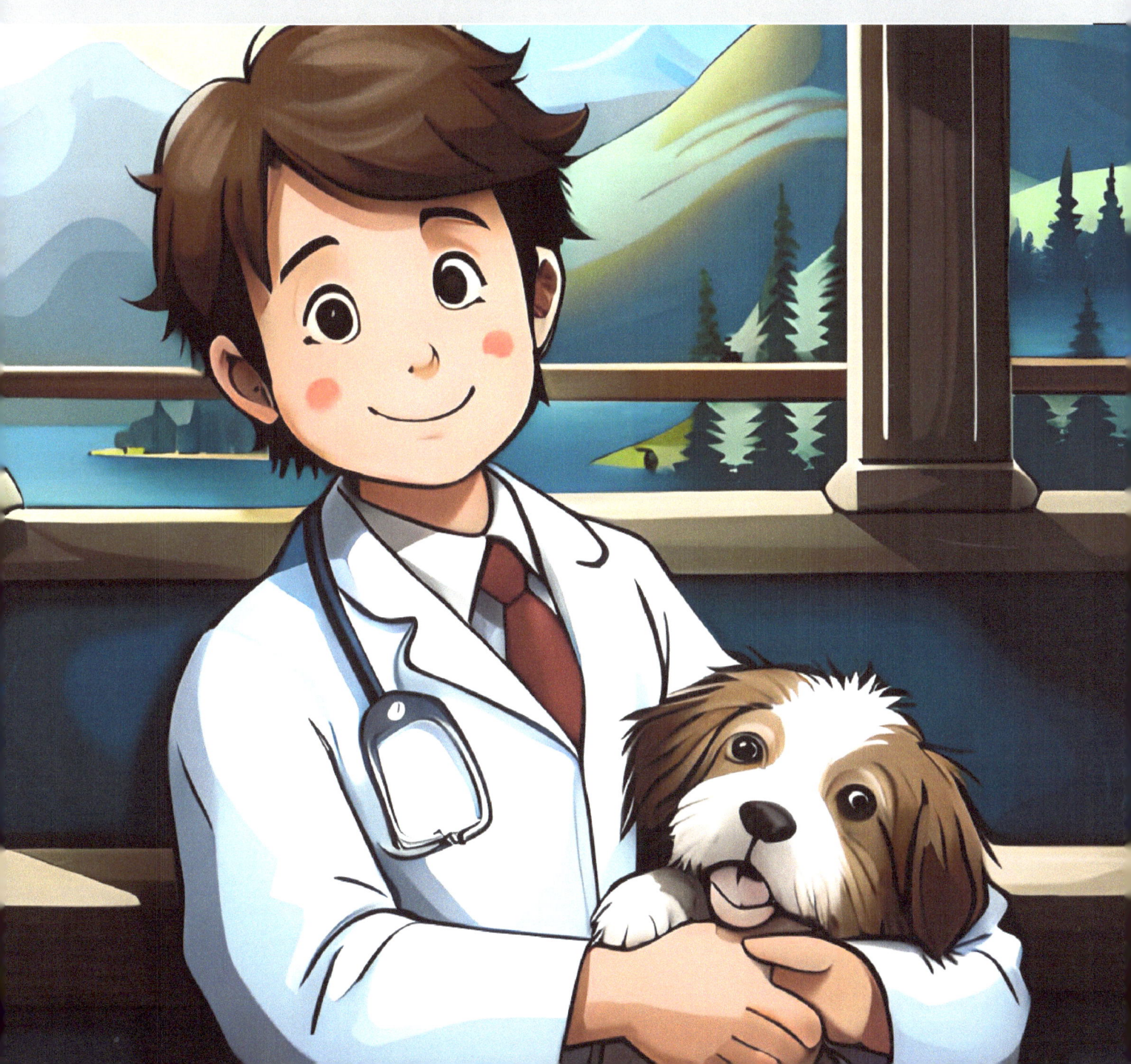

As Little Vet continued to explore the world of veterinary medicine, he began to wonder how he could become a veterinarian himself. He learned that it would take many years of education and training to become a licensed veterinarian.

The Little Vet discovered that he would need to complete an undergraduate degree in a relevant field, such as biology, animal science or pre-veterinary studies..

In veterinary school, the Little Vet would study a wide range of subjects, including anatomy, physiology, pharmacology and surgery. He would also have to complete clinical internships and gain hands-on experience working with animals in various settings.

Little Vet learned that becoming a veterinarian requires not only a strong academic background, but also strong interpersonal skills. Compassion, empathy and effective communication are important when working with animals and their owners.

The young vet knew that the road ahead would be challenging, but he was determined to follow his dreams and become a veterinarian. He was excited to learn all he could about this amazing profession and help animals and their owners in any way he could.

In pursuit of a lifelong dream,
The little veterinarian began to scheme,
To learn about animals big and small,
And how to heal them, one and all.

They started with basics of pet care,
Nutrition, hygiene, and exercise to share,
Then moved on to anatomy and more,
Learning about each body system's core.

Surgery and emergency care they studied too,
Knowing these skills could save a pet or two,
And rehabilitation for those in need,
To help animals heal and again succeed.

Specializations in the field they explored,
Exotic animals, marine mammals, they adored,
And the different roles within the vet team,
Vet techs, assistants, and behaviorists supreme.

Finally, the time had come to learn,
How to become a vet, with great concern,
Years of study and hard work lay ahead,
But with passion and drive, they'd forge ahead.

The little veterinarian was ready to take flight,
To help animals with all their might,
To care for them with empathy and grace,
And make the world a better place.

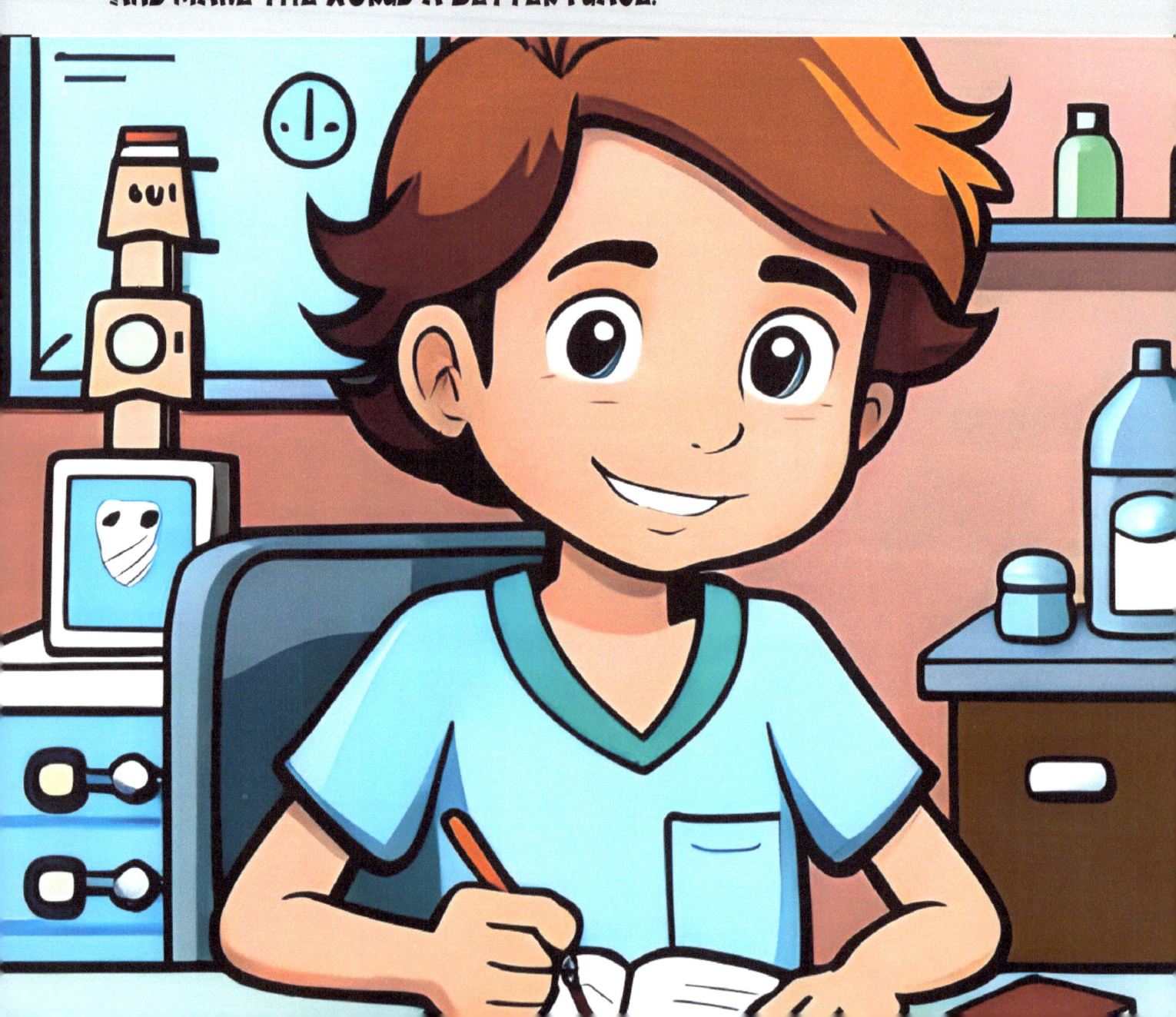

Chapter 9: The Little Veterinarian in Action

The little veterinarian was excited to put their knowledge and skills to work in the community. They started by volunteering at a local animal shelter, where they helped care for the cats and dogs waiting for their forever homes. They cleaned cages, fed the animals, and took them for walks and playtime.

As they got more involved with the shelter, the little veterinarian noticed some of the animals had health issues that needed attention. They spoke to the shelter staff and offered to use their skills to help. With permission from the shelter veterinarian, they were able to provide basic care like cleaning wounds and administering medication.

Word quickly spread about the little veterinarian's skills, and soon they were being asked to help out at other shelters and rescue organizations in the area. They also started providing basic pet care and education to their neighbors, helping to keep pets healthy and happy in their own homes.

The little veterinarian felt fulfilled by their work in the community and knew that they had found their calling. They dreamed of one day opening their own veterinary practice, where they could continue to make a difference in the lives of animals and their owners.

As the little veterinarian helped the animals in need,
They found a purpose, a cause to heed.
With every wound they cleaned and every pill they gave,
They felt a sense of purpose that they couldn't waive.

At the shelter, they worked with cats and dogs,
Cleaning their cages and taking them for long walks.
They gave them love and care, and soon they could see,
That these animals were happier than they used to be.

Then one day, they noticed a dog with a limp,
And they knew that they had to act in a quick blip.
They spoke to the staff and offered to help,
And soon they were treating animals with yelps and yelps.

Word of their skills soon spread around,
And more people came, animals to be found.
The little veterinarian worked hard day and night,
Providing care to animals with all their might.

They dreamt of one day owning their own clinic,
Where they could help even more animals, no limit.
They knew it would take time, hard work, and dedication,
But they were ready for the challenge, no hesitation.

CHAPTER 10: THE LITTLE VETERINARIAN'S FUTURE

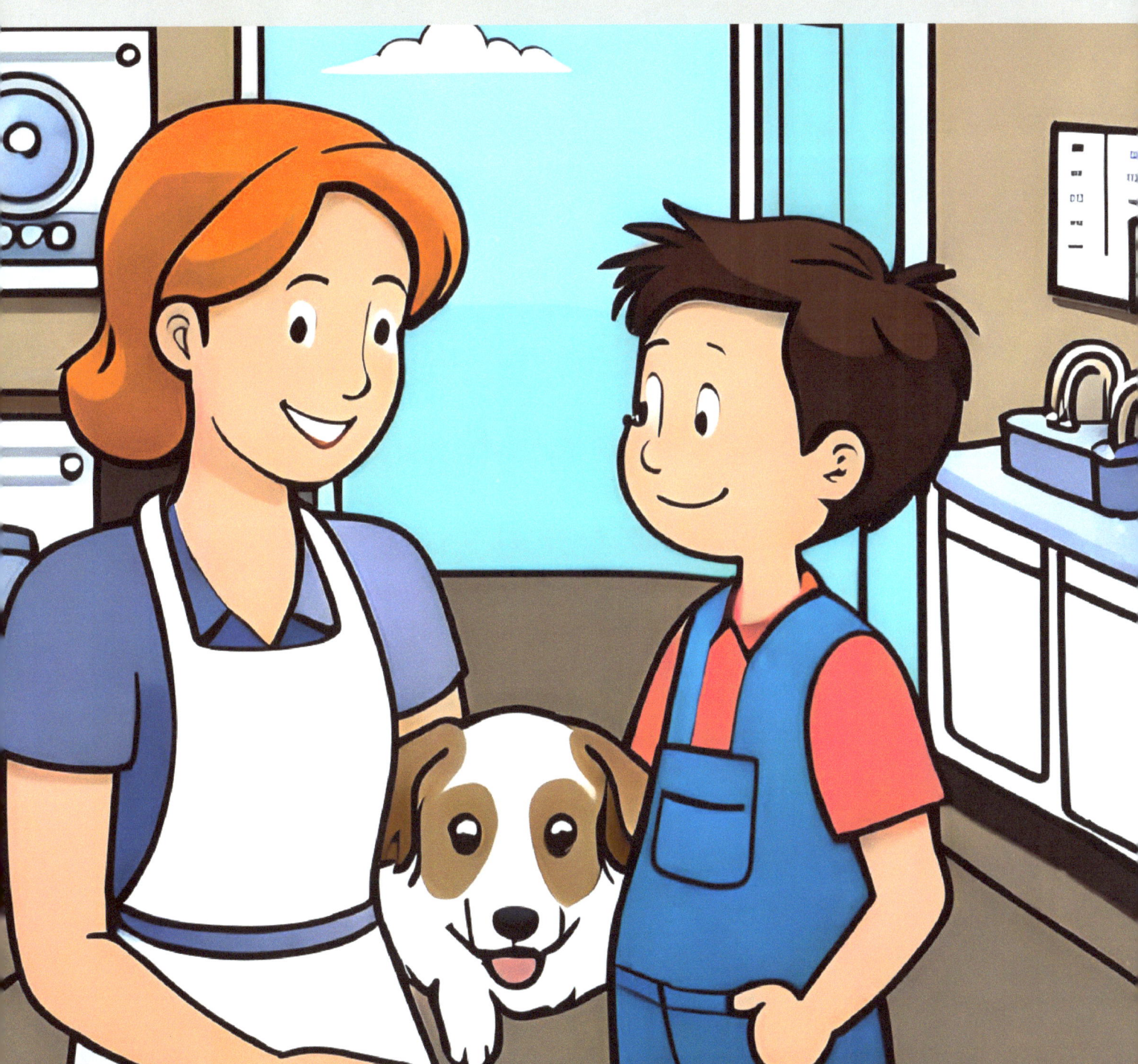

As the little veterinarian grew older and wiser,
They continued to strive and never tired.
Their love for animals remained strong,
And they knew they wanted to do nothing wrong.

They thought about their dreams and what they wanted to achieve,
And knew that their goals they couldn't leave.
They dreamed of opening their own clinic one day,
Where they could provide care in their own special way.

They knew it would take time, hard work, and a lot of grit,
But they were determined and wouldn't quit.
They continued to study and learn every day,
And worked with animals in every possible way.

And as they looked back on their journey so far,
They knew they had come very far.
They had helped so many animals, big and small,
And knew they had answered their calling, answering the call.

And so, with their dreams and goals set high,
The little veterinarian continued to reach for the sky.
They knew that they had a bright future ahead,
And that they would continue to help animals until the end.

Once upon a time, in a far-off land,
There was a little girl with a veterinarian plan.
She loved all animals, big and small,
And knew she wanted to help them all.

She studied hard and learned a lot,
About animal care and the health they sought.
She dreamed of becoming a veterinarian,
To help animals who were sick or hurt again and again.

With each passing day, she grew more skilled,
And knew that one day, her dreams would be fulfilled.
She practiced her skills with every chance,
And worked with animals at every glance.

One day, a sick kitten came her way,
And she knew she had to save the day.
She examined the kitten with care,
And knew just what she had to repair.

With her knowledge and skills in tow,
She gave the kitten the care it needed to grow.
And when the kitten was finally well,
The little girl knew her calling quite well.

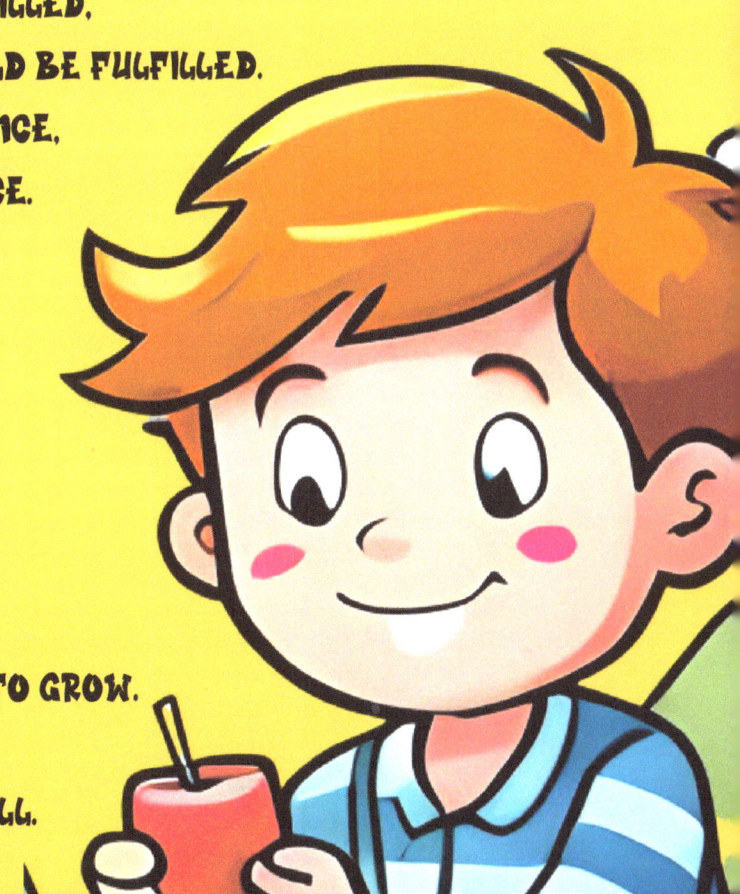

She continued to study and learn more,
About animal care, down to the core.
And as she grew older and wiser too,
Her dreams and passions only grew.

She worked with animals far and wide,
And always had a smile by her side.
For she knew that her calling was true,
And that helping animals was all she wanted to do.

And so, the little girl with a veterinarian plan,
Became a skilled vet, with knowledge in her hand.
She helped animals big and small,
And knew she was answering her calling, once and for all.

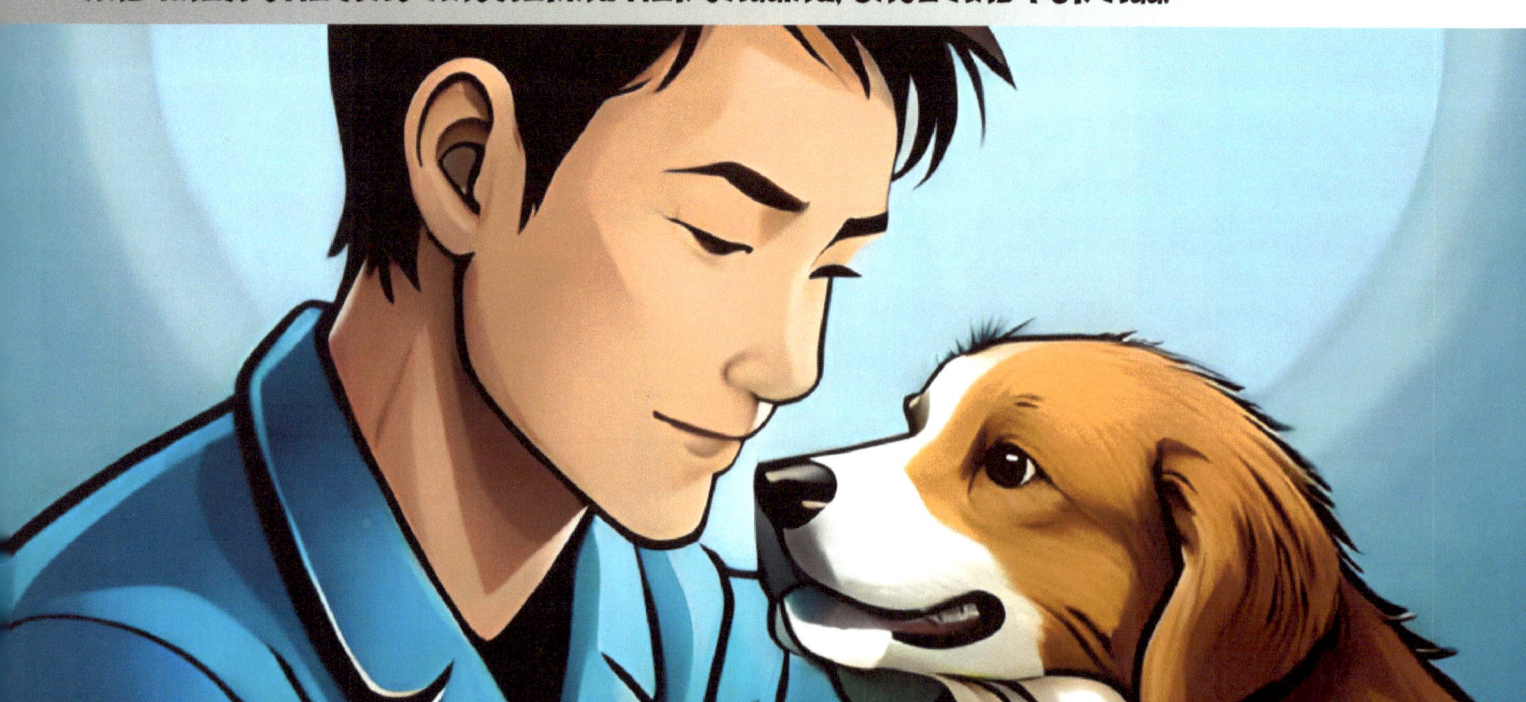

www.ingramcontent.com/pod-product-compliance
Lightning Source LLC
Chambersburg PA
CBHW040410220526

45473CB00004B/1195